W9-BTQ-952

SHIATSU

ABOUT THE AUTHORS

From the age of 14 Chris Jarmey has studied and practised Hatha Yoga and a variety of martial arts. He has been studying, practising and subsequently teaching Shiatsu since 1970, drawing mainly upon the inspirations of Shizuto Masunaga, and more recently Michael Rose and Pauline Sasaki. After qualifying in physiotherapy in 1978, and becoming a state registered physiotherapist, he initiated the use of both Shiatsu and therapeutic yoga methods into the hospital environment. Having created a teaching network throughout England and Wales for 'grassroots' Shiatsu, he founded the Shiatsu School of Natural Therapy in 1985 as a vehicle for teaching Shiatsu up to practitioner level. The school has since expanded to become the European Shiatsu School with several branches throughout Britain and Europe. Chris is the Principal of the European Shiatsu School, and sits on the Core Group and Examining Board of the Shiatsu Society. He is also the Medical Liaison Officer and correspondent for the Society.

Gabriel Mojay is a qualified and experienced Shiatsu practitioner and a registered member of the Shiatsu Society. He has also been trained in acupuncture, and is a member of the Traditional Acupuncture Society. A qualified medical herbalist, he is Assistant Director of the Institute of Traditional Herbal Medicine and Aromatherapy. He has a private practice in Shiatsu, acupuncture, medical herbalism and aromatherapy. Since 1983 Gabriel has taught a variety of approaches to natural healing, including oriental medicine and Shiatsu in particular.

SHIATSU
The complete guide

Chris Jarmey and Gabriel Mojay

Illustrated by Peter Cox
Photography by Peter Warren

Thorsons
An Imprint of HarperCollins*Publishers*

Thorsons
An Imprint of HarperCollins*Publishers*
77–85 Fulham Palace Road
Hammersmith, London W6 8JB

Published by Thorsons 1991
7 9 10 8 6

© Chris Jarmey and Gabriel Mojay 1991

Chris Jarmey and Gabriel Mojay assert the moral
right to be identified as the authors of this work

A catalogue record for this book
is available from the British Library

ISBN 0 7225 2243 6

Typeset by Burns & Smith Limited
Printed in Great Britain by The Bath Press, Bath, Avon

Contents

A NOTE ON THE USE OF CAPITALIZATION

Throughout this book you will notice that all words referring to concepts peculiar to Oriental Medicine begin with a capital letter. When the same words describe a more familiar western meaning, they do not. This is standard practice to avoid misrepresentation of meaning. For example, 'Liver' refers to the Oriental medical concept of Liver, whereas 'liver' refers to the anatomical liver organ as understood in western medicine. Other words used in this book such as: Heat, Full, Channel and so on, all have slightly different connotations in Oriental Medicine.

Introduction

WHAT IS SHIATSU?

Shiatsu is a form of bodywork which, at its highest level, combines a finely-tuned intuition with a thorough understanding of the bodymind. Shiatsu was developed in Japan from a synthesis of Chinese massage called Anma and Western techniques of physical manipulation. As a complete system of healing through touch, it draws extensively on key aspects of Traditional Oriental Medicine.

Shiatsu technique involves stretching, holding and leaning body weight into various part of the recipient's body to improve energy flow, blood circulation, flexibility and posture. Pressure and contact is applied through the hands, thumbs, fingers, forearms, knees and feet, with the recipient sitting or lying in various positions. Treatment is focused along specific Channels ('meridians') of subtle bodily energy called Ki. Ki is the life force which sustains every activity of the body, mind and Spirit.

Although Shiatsu literally means 'finger pressure', the spirit of Shiatsu is one of communication through touch. Shiatsu which is responsive to the recipient's needs cannot be achieved by technical skill and intellectual study alone. To be effective, it requires sensitivity in order to feel and positively influence the quality of vitality within the recipient. Vitality is the basis of health, and reflects the strength and harmony of Ki circulation. Shiatsu which is sensitive and supportive both tonifies and corrects the flow of Ki, thereby helping to restore vitality and prevent disease.

To achieve truly supportive Shiatsu, it must be delivered with relaxed body weight and an effortless transmission of Ki. Overt effort from the practitioner will only obstruct Ki flow and prevent the recipient from relaxing and 'opening'. Ki is naturally communicated to the recipient when the practitioner's energy is focused and 'grounded' in the lower belly (the belly is referred to as 'the hara' by Shiatsu practitioners).

Finally, truly accurate Shiatsu therapy depends upon the practitioner's understanding of Traditional Oriental Medicine and its diagnostic skills. A practitioner who is knowledgable will have sufficient confidence to deal with clients suffering from both acute and chronic disorders.

THE HISTORY OF SHIATSU

Although the word Shiatsu was not coined until the early twentieth century, the origins of Shiatsu lie firmly within the roots of Traditional Oriental Medicine. Specifically, it can be traced to China around 530 BC, when Bodhidharma introduced a system of exercises for health and sensory control known as Tao-Yinn. These incorporated a system of self-massage and self-applied pressure point therapy for promoting detoxification and rejuvenation. Tao-Yinn soon became an integral part of the health practices and was gradually exported, along with the other Chinese healing arts, through south-east Asia and Korea.

By the tenth century AD, Chinese Medicine had been introduced into Japan, from which time an amalgam of Vibrational Palm Healing, Spot Pressing and Massage, known collectively as Anma, would have been combined with Tao-Yinn (Do-In) to loosely resemble present day Shiatsu.

Around three hundred years ago, during the Edo era in Japan, doctors were required to study Anma as a means of familiarizing themselves with the human structure, energy channels and pressure points, so that they could accurately diagnose and treat with whatever means they thought appropriate; namely acupuncture, herbs or bodywork. Gradually, however, Anma was reduced to treating simple muscular tensions until by the twentieth century it became licensed only to promote pleasure and comfort.

However, there still existed many Anma therapists who based their work on the original theory, and who coined the name Shiatsu in order to avoid the restrictive regulations applied to Anma. Shiatsu was eventually recognized as a legitimate form of therapy by the Japanese government in the mid-1950s.

Nowadays the official definition given by the Japanese Ministry of Health and Welfare states:

> Shiatsu therapy is a form of manipulation administered by the thumbs, fingers and palms, without the use of any instrument, mechanical or otherwise, to apply pressure to the human skin, to correct internal malfunctioning, promote and maintain health and treat specific diseases.

The Development of Shiatsu in Japan

The official recognition of Shiatsu in Japan can be mainly attributed to the efforts of Tokujiro Namikoshi, who established the Shiatsu Institute of Therapy in Hokkaido in 1925 and the Japan Shiatsu Institute in 1940 (subsequently renamed the Japan Shiatsu School). His success was no doubt due to a combination of his obvious tactile sensitivity and the effort he put into aligning Shiatsu with Western medicine. In this way, his method benefited from the general trend towards Westernization.

The traditional, philosophical and medical framework was reintegrated into Shiatsu by Shizuto Masunaga, who taught at the Japan Shiatsu Institute for ten years before opening his own school known as the Iokai Shiatsu Centre in Tokyo. Also highly developed in tactile sensitivity, Shizuto Masunaga had an interest in integrating the ancient medical model with Western physiology. His main contribution to Shiatsu before his death was to establish the full influence of the major Energy Channels over the surface of the body, and how to fully effect a person's psychological/physical balance through optimum connection with these Channels.

Consequently, in Japan today, there are two distinct methods of Shiatsu: the method developed by Tokujiro Namikoshi, and Iokai Shiatsu as developed by the late Shizuto Masunaga. Namikoshi's style is characterized by applying pressure to specific reflex points which relate to the central and autonomic nervous system, whereas Masunaga's style is characterized by sensitivity to the Energy Channels which are the manifestation of body/mind function, from the viewpoint of Oriental Medicine. Masunaga also introduced the dimension of 'support and connection' by realizing that Shiatsu treatment is much less painful, more nurturing and energetically more effective if both hands are kept apart, yet in contact with the recipient, so that one hand is used as a 'listening' hand, while the other applies technique.

Between the two polarities, there are several Japanese acupuncture schools which teach Shiatsu as a prerequisite to studying acupuncture. Ultimately, however, the effectiveness of Shiatsu depends more upon the attitude, proficiency and attunement of the practitioner, than upon a particular style.

The Development of Shiatsu in the West

Shiatsu did not become widely known in the United States and Europe until the 1970s, although it has been practised by a few Japanese and Occidentals in the West since its conception. Within Europe, Shiatsu has been primarily influenced by the Namikoshi method and the Masunaga method, but with an additional input from macrobiotics[1] which makes use of the traditional Acupuncture Channels and pressure points, plus its own theoretical and philosophical rationale. This method incorporates substantial use of the feet to apply pressure and stretch, commonly known as 'Barefoot' techniques. Shiatsu as practised in Europe is therefore mostly associated with either Masunaga's method (often called Zen Shiatsu), Macrobiotic Shiatsu, Namikoshi method, or various hybrids.

In the United States, Shiatsu had – by the mid 1980s – been classified into the following systems or 'styles':

- *Acupressure Shiatsu*, which focuses specifically upon acupuncture points and encompasses a variety of acupressure styles.
- *Five Element Style Shiatsu*, which relies mainly upon the Five

Element Theory[2] of Traditional Chinese Medicine, especially in relation to the emotions, and which incorporates some macrobiotic principles.

- *Macrobiotic Shiatsu*, which incorporates Classical Acupuncture Channels, Barefoot techniques and the way of living in harmony as advocated by George Ohsawa, Michio Kushi and others.
- *Nippon Style Shiatsu*, which is fundamentally Namikoshi style, and as such places great emphasis on Western physiology, but with the addition of Chinese medical theory and the Classical Energy Channels.
- *Zen Shiatsu*, as developed by Shizuto Masunaga, which is characterized by the application of the Kyo-Jitsu Tonification and Sedation Principle,[3] an extended Energy Channel system, and a condensed synthesis of Traditional Chinese Medicine, Western physiology and psychology.
- *Ohashiatsu*, can also be added to this list as an amalgam of Namikoshi's style with methods developed by Wataru Ohashi, aspects of Zen Shiatsu, and the use of Classical acupoints (Tsubos) and Channels.

It is interesting to observe that in Japan, which has traditionally enjoyed a rich heritage of Traditional Chinese Medicine, the most popular method of Shiatsu first licensed by the Japanese government was the Namikoshi system, which is based upon Western medical concepts to the exclusion of all Traditional Chinese Medical theory and Energy Channels.

Conversely, in both Europe and the United States, all styles of Shiatsu, including those derived from the Namikoshi method, incorporate some aspect of Traditional Oriental Medicine.

1. Macrobiotics is a philosophy of living and eating for harmony and self-development, systemized by George Ohsawa.
2. The Five Elements are fully described in Chapter 10 of this book.
3. Kyo-Jitsu is described extensively throughout this book, see particularly pp.17–19.

PART 1

THE BASICS OF SHIATSU

Shiatsu is a method of bodywork which allows us to give and receive care, warmth and healing through non-intrusive touch. Its potential role within society is forever increasing as we become more divorced from direct personal communication and tactile human contact. Within our industrialized, technological age, there exists a move towards greater human connection and co-operation; Shiatsu will greatly facilitate this.

In this section we will present the basics of Shiatsu necessary to fulfil this need at an appropriate level for use amongst family and friends. These basic principles are, however, equally applicable to Shiatsu as a therapy, and as such should be considered the foundation to Shiatsu practice at all levels.

To appreciate fully the power of Shiatsu, it is necessary at the outset to understand the Oriental concept of energy and its inter-relationship with the human being. To this end, we will firstly define Ki, Channels and Tsubos, and then highlight the difference in emphasis between acupressure and Shiatsu, with a description of Kyo/Jitsu.

Chapter 1

The Concept of Ki

WHAT IS KI?

The difference between that which is living and that which is not living is the relative quantity of what oriental medical tradition speaks of as *Ki* and *Jing*. Ki (Chinese Qi or Ch'i) can be thought of as the power which unifies and animates. It binds energy into matter, which means that without it nothing would hold together and nothing tangible would exist. Ki is therefore a binding, cohesive force at the point where energy is on the verge of materializing, and where matter is at the point of becoming energy. Since matter is itself a form of energy vibration, everything in existence is considered to be Ki. However, it makes for clearer understanding if we limit our interpretation of Ki to be that which animates matter. Therefore beyond its fundamental binding qualities, Ki is also the energy associated with any movement, be it the movement of the sea, wind, blood or of walking. All inanimate and animate things must therefore have Ki to exist, and more Ki to move.

In order to 'live', however, an organism must pass through a process of organic change ranging from birth and growth towards eventual decay. The life essence which makes this possible is known as *Jing* or *Essence*. Jing therefore, is the source of living substance and growth whereas Ki is the ability to bind, activate and move.

However, an organism can exist with sufficient Jing to fulfil its involuntary organic processes and have enough Ki to function, without necessarily exhibiting an indication of consciousness. Consciousness signifies the presence of *Shen*, which is the energy behind the power to think and discriminate, to rationalize and to self reflect. Without Shen, there can be no personality. Ki, Jing and Shen are known in traditional oriental thinking as 'the three Treasures'.

Ki is more widespread than Jing or Shen, because everything we perceive (and much that we do not) has some degree of Ki. Only that which is 'living' in the sense that it is subject to growth, reproduction and decay, has Jing. Only that which is conscious and can self reflect (e.g. humans) has Shen. It is important to realize that Jing and Shen are limited aspects or special manifestations of Ki, as is everything else that exists. Reference to Ki henceforth will refer to its functional aspects of cohesion and movement.

All matter, or in fact anything we can conceptualize, be it a thought or an emotion, has Ki. The difference between the living and the non-living is the presence of Jing, to which Shen may add consciousness. However, Jing and Shen cannot manifest without the cohesive and moving attributes of Ki. The more alive you are, the more Ki you have. An abundance of Ki in a living organism results in high vitality. If a person lacks vitality they will lack the optimum quota of Ki to infuse the Jing and Shen. If they are dead, they are very deficient in Ki (and devoid of Jing and Shen). Decomposition reflects a further depletion until the only Ki remaining is the *minimum* needed to keep the atoms and molecules manifesting as matter. Ki will not produce life, but life is impossible without sufficient Ki.

Ki is everywhere, on and around this earth, although some places have more than others. Moving water generates Ki in abundance, whilst Ki itself is the ultimate source of that movement. This presence of Ki can clearly be appreciated in the proximity of waterfalls and by the sea-shore.

Sunlight is undoubtedly the greatest source of Ki from our perspect-ive. The level of Ki necessary to charge matter with life cannot occur in the absence of sunlight or water. This is obvious with plants, but equally true of animals who can only exist by eating plants or other animals, who themselves feed on plants. Even fungi, which seem to flourish without direct access to sunlight, grow out of material produced by the plants and animals which do.

Sources of Ki in the Body

In order for 'life' to be maintained within our bodies, we must have a constant input of Ki to keep things together and moving. This input is from 3 main sources; initially we inherit it from parents and subsequently we obtain it from air and food. Ki will be explained in greater detail in its relationship to specific oriental medical theory in Part 2 of this book.

WHAT IS A CHANNEL?

Channels – or meridians – are said to be the routes through which Ki flows, forming a network connecting up the Ki associated with all the major functions of the body. The concept of interconnecting Channels is termed *Jing Luo* in Traditional Oriental Medicine. *Jing*[1] means 'to go', 'steer through' or 'to direct', and *Luo* means 'a net', 'network' or 'an attaching system'. We consider *Jing Luo* to carry Ki to all the tissues and organs, whereas Blood is carried within the blood vessels (known as *Xue Mai*). Traditionally, however, the carriage of Ki and Blood within Channels and blood vessels was not precisely differentiated because the

Channels were considered to carry Ki *and* Blood, and blood vessels were considered to carry Blood *and* Ki. To avoid confusion, it is easier to consider the Channels as carrying *only* Ki, although it must be remembered that Ki is the force behind all movement, including the movement of Blood which means that Ki exists in abundance in the blood vessels. Channels can be thought of as 'carrying' Blood in the sense that where the Ki within the Channels is felt to be deficient in a particular body area, there is often an accompanying lack of blood circulation.

Blood vessels and nerves are easy to define because they can be 'seen' to exist, from their precise location upon dissection of the body. We cannot in the same way locate the Channels, which implies they have no physical structure, and do not exist within a dead body.[2] Unlike the electrical wiring of a house which exists whether or not electricity is flowing through it, Channels do not exist independently of Ki. A good comparison is that a beam cannot exist without light. It must be that a Channel and its Ki are one and the same, and exist or cease to exist according to the presence or absence of life.

To help conceptualize a Channel, an analogy can be drawn with water currents. A body of water such as the sea may have specific currents of water flowing through it as a consequence of feeder streams, tidal movements and thermals. However, if the source of these currents is removed by blocking the feeder streams and equalizing the water temperatures throughout, then the course of the deceased water current becomes undetectable. Likewise, the cessation of living functions remove the source of a Channel's existence. A dead body, therefore, has no Ki Channels,[2] in the same way that it has no soul or personality.

You can of course, map out where the surface course of the Channels 'should be' or 'once were' by drawing lines all over the body to match diagrammatic charts. However, this can encourage a 'static' concept of Channel location. In actuality, a Channel's Ki strength and quality will be affected by bodily disharmonies, and its precise location will slightly alter according to variations in Ki flow within adjacent Channels. Again, we can compare this with a water current whose precise location may be altered by variable activity within nearby currents.

Since a Channel may not be quite where it 'should be' according to the map, and since variable factors will alter the exact angle of touch necessary to connect with the Ki, it is essential for the Shiatsu practitioner to develop sensitivity to the continuity of Ki flow in order to maximize the effect of the Shiatsu session.

WHAT IS A TSUBO?

A *Tsubo* is any point along the surface pathway of a Ki Channel where the Ki can be influenced directly by pressure, or by needle insertion. Tsubos are gateways into a person's energetic body and as such, they

Fig. 1.1: Tsubo
The character represents a jar with a narrow neck covered with a lid. The neck represents the Tsubo connecting to the Ki within the Channel represented by the bulbous section of the jar.

can be used to affect the internal environment of a human being.

Acupuncture makes use of those points which have fixed locations. Since they are fixed, these points, when manipulated, have actions on the body and mind which have been recorded empirically for many centuries. A Tsubo does not have to be a fixed and labelled point however, and Shiatsu makes use of those Tsubos which manifest along the Channels *between* the fixed points, as well as the fixed points themselves.

Fixed Tsubos are both energetic vortices where the *normal* or *constant* life processes are relayed to the surface, and where there is an intake or release of Ki between the Channels and the outside world. In contrast, the non-fixed Tsubos are surface reflections of *fluctuating* functional imbalances. The experienced Shiatsu practitioner is able to detect these Tsubos as palpable distortions in the Ki flow of the Channels. In so doing, energy can be tonified if weak, dispersed if in excess or blocked, and calmed if over active, according to the method of touch applied.

Tsubos cannot exist without Ki any more than their Channels can. Both are reactions to the internal environment which is constantly influencing Ki strength and circulation. The energetic outline of a Tsubo is like a vase-shaped vortice with its mouth and neck narrower than its base. The Japanese character for Tsubo illustrates this shape quite accurately.

The experienced Shiatsu practitioner is able to feel the depth and breadth of a Tsubo and feel its response to touch. Also, since everything in the body is connected in some way to everything else, he or she is able to feel resultant reactions in other Tsubos elsewhere in the body.

THE DIFFERENCE BETWEEN SHIATSU AND ACUPRESSURE

Shiatsu can be applied evenly or with variable pressure along the length of Ki Channels. Pressure applied evenly and rhythmically has a smoothing effect on the Ki flow, whereas variable yet stationary pressure, applied according to the level of Ki within the non-fixed Tsubos, will have a deeper effect, because it requires greater focus from the giver.

Most Shiatsu systems are based upon tactile connection with the Ki flowing within the Channels. An exception is the Namikoshi system in Japan which uses neuromuscular physiology as its theoretical basis. Methods which concentrate on the classical 'fixed' Tsubos for their specific reactions upon the body and mind are known as Acupressure. In contrast, Shiatsu focuses less upon the classical Tsubos and more upon the Channel pathways themselves.

Acupressure is generally geared to relieving the recipient's suffering by tonifying weak Ki, calming overactive Ki, or dispersing blocked Ki via the classical Tsubos. Systems which emphasize the classical Tsubos often view deficient Ki as an independent phenomenon from excess Ki, and vice versa. Shiatsu differs in so far as it deals more with the interaction between Ki Channels, viewing excess or deficiency as distortions in the energetic web of Ki flow. Therefore it is recognized that excess Ki within one Tsubo often requires a relative deficiency within another. If a Channel has predominantly excess Ki, then another must be relatively deficient. Channel imbalances are therefore seen as reflecting relative distortions within the person as a whole. Shiatsu is based upon rectifying Channel distortions. However, most Shiatsu systems incorporate some acupressure technique.

KYO JITSU

Assessing and balancing interacting Channel distortions is highly developed in the Zen Shiatsu system. Shizuto Masunaga referred to depleted, empty or underactive Ki as *Kyo*, and excess, full or hyperactive Ki as *Jitsu*. Both Kyo and Jitsu refer to relative states of emptiness and fullness, and therefore do not exist or mean anything in the absence of the other. Masunaga draws the analogy of Kyo/Jitsu distortion with vector distortions in a ball. From Fig. 1.2 we can see that the empty, depressed Kyo area gives rise to the full, protruding Jitsu area.

You can expect any Channel to err towards Kyo or Jitsu in relation to any other. The whole pattern is constantly fluctuating. The aim of Shiatsu is to discover the root cause behind any acute or chronic disharmony and attempt to stabilize it. The Jitsu areas are easy to find because they exhibit activity and protrude from the surface. They are however, only the result of deeper weakness, less obviously exhibited as Kyo elsewhere.

The most direct and surest way to balance overall Kyo/Jitsu distortions and therefore allow the body/mind its optimum potential for healing is to find the most Kyo Channel and balance it off against the Channel which is most Jitsu. All the other minor imbalances in the other Channels will tend to equalize as a result.

The emptying or moving of Jitsu is referred to as *sedation* or *dispersal*, whereas the filling and strengthening of Kyo is referred to as *tonification*. It is essential that Kyo/Jitsu is accurately assessed, and that a recipient who is generally weak is not further weakened by the overuse of dispersal techniques. This can easily occur because Jitsu is much easier to locate within the body than Kyo. Each Channel exhibits differing degrees of Kyo/Jitsu emphasis throughout its own pathway, so that once the most Kyo and most Jitsu Channels have been located, each must be dealt with according to their energetic presentation. The most profound part of a treatment will be the tonification of the weakest Tsubos within the weakest area of the weakest Channel.

The principle methods of tonifying Kyo and dispersing Jitsu are fully explained in Chapter 3 (p.34).

Fig. 1.2: Kyo/Jitsu

Comparison of Kyo/Jitsu

Kyo	Jitsu
Below surface	Protruding from surface
Less obvious	More obvious
Passive resistance or no resistance	Active resistance
Empty – requires filling	Full – requires emptying/dispersing
Underactive, leading to stiffness or flaccidity	Hyperactive, leading to congestion, blockage and impenetrability
Slower to respond	Immediate response
Underlying cause	Manifests as symptoms
Requires deep, sustained connection	Requires light, superficial connection, or none at all
Its tonification affects the whole person	Its dispersal affects localized body areas

Both Kyo and Jitsu can feel hard and unyielding to touch, which can confuse the inexperienced practitioner. Kyo can have the impenetrable feeling of a solid, locked door to an empty room. The impenetrability of Jitsu, however, is analogous to the sheer volume of people within a room who can do without your presence to add to the squeeze. Ki however, is more tenuous than crowds of people, so it takes a degree of subtlety and awareness to detect its measure.

A useful analogy can be drawn from knocking on the doors of houses in a street:

a. Some reveal an obvious presence because someone answers the door (Ki is clearly present);
b. The person who answers the door may aggressively send you away (Extreme Jitsu);
c. They may open the door before you knock and send you away (Very extreme Jitsu);
d. Someone opens the door out of curiosity and allows you into the lobby, if you are pleasant to them (Neutral);
e. Someone answers the door, is lonely and desperate for company, so encourages you to come in (Acute Kyo);
f. Nobody is in and the door is wide open (Flaccid Kyo);
g. Nobody is in, but the door is double-bolted for security (Chronic stiff Kyo).

From this analogy we can see that the attitude and approach of the caller is important. A very aggressive caller (or Shiatsu technique) might succeed in forcing their way in where they are not welcome, causing pain and a great deal of discord in the neighbourhood (which is analogous to the body/mind). The same caller might overstep the hospitality of those desperate for company, causing tension as a defensive reaction. A particularly insensitive and aggressive 'caller' might smash down the bolted door to get 'results' and thus cause permanent damage.

Aggression and insensitivity are therefore the antithesis of gaining safe and welcome entry into both house and Tsubo. Sensitivity and patience is required in all circumstances.

Recognizing degrees of deficiency within the chronic stiff Kyo areas requires almost ethereal subtlety. It can be done quite easily with practice if you again think of Ki within a Tsubo as similar to people within a house. When you knock on enough doors you develop a sense of *knowing* when nobody is in, or when somebody is *pretending* not to be in, even though both seem to be empty at first glance. In Kyo Tsubos you are therefore tuning your senses to the detection of a presence, even if it does not want to show itself. When you have found it, you can offer it your support.

1. *Jing* – not to be confused with the term 'Jing' meaning 'Essence' in another context.
2. Channels, however, do seem to affect the tissues through which they pass, with changes that persist even after death. Research in China led by Professor Zhu Zong Xiang from Beijing shows that the skin is thinner along the Channels than it is adjacent to them. He also discovered that infrasonic waves travel more quickly and with a higher pitch along Channel pathways than in surrounding areas. Professor Zhang Baozhen has also found that nerve endings are more expanded along the course of major Channels compared to elsewhere.

Chapter 2

The Essentials of Competent Shiatsu

The basic aims of Shiatsu for use at a grassroots level amongst family and friends are:

- To help the recipient relax and therefore provide a means to combat the effects of stress;
- To improve the recipient's lymphatic flow, blood circulation and vitality (and therefore boost the immune system);
- To help alleviate aches, pains and stiffness;
- To help both the giver and receiver become more aware of their bodies;
- To develop healing compassion through appropriate physical contact.

These aims are most readily achieved if the giver of Shiatsu applies the essential ingredients of Shiatsu, which are:

- Motivation
- Steadiness of breath
- Strong and open Hara
- Relaxation and comfort
- Empty Mind
- Support rather than force
- Positive connection

- Perpendicular pressure
- Stationary pressure
- Technical ability
- Continuity
- Fluency
- Empathy

MOTIVATION

To give Shiatsu there must be a genuine desire to help people feel better. If this desire is absent then there can be no sincere motivation for being involved with this humanitarian healing art.

It is interesting that the written character for 'human' in Japanese embodies the Shiatsu qualities of support and connection, which are fundamental qualities of the human ideal.

You will find that giving Shiatsu makes you feel better, more grounded and more open both physically and energetically, because the more you give of yourself in the service of humankind, the more universal Ki will come flooding back in. This is because nature hates empty spaces. The motivation for giving Shiatsu should be to help others, thereby helping yourself.

Fig. 2.1: The Japanese Character for Human; each stem is clearly supporting the other. Mutual support is achieved by leaning and relaxing rather than tensing and pushing

STEADINESS OF BREATH

The breath is intimately connected to thought processes, insofar as deep relaxed breathing produces equanimity of mind and vice versa. Scattered, unfocused thoughts are usually reflected in shallow, irregular breathing, whereas focused attention of the mind only manifests when the breath has slowed to a point where there is a natural period of 'no breathing' between exhalation and inhalation. This can be demonstrated by asking someone to drop a pin somewhere out of sight but within earshot. Listening for the almost imperceptible sound of the pin drop requires such focused attention that the breath stops momentarily. The ability to listen for a pin drop amongst intense distractions fighting for the attention of the mind and emotions is an example of being 'centred'. Centredness is therefore proportional to steadiness of breath, while erratic, shallow breath is symptomatic of those who are not grounded. For the giver of Shiatsu, being 'centred' means being able to feel the barely perceptible changes in muscle tone, circulation and energy levels, as well as having the sensitivity to tune into the recipient's frame of mind; it is knowing when the recipient's tensions relax both physically and mentally. One is truly centred if all this can be achieved irrespective of ongoing personal conflicts and all other distractions.

STRONG AND OPEN HARA

Increased centredness can be achieved in many ways. Most spiritual disciplines, if they are practised sincerely, will be of great value, but more especially if there is some emphasis on drawing the mind to the belly, which is the actual physical centre of the body, known as the *Hara*. The energetic centre and physical pivot point of the Hara is known as the *Tanden*, which is located below the navel in the lower abdomen. Aikido, Qi-Qong, Tai-Chi, Yoga, Zen and various meditation methods are all excellent for developing Hara strength and awareness. Focusing energy in the Hara harmonizes the body, mind emotions and spirit, which enables us to harmonize with our surroundings and to react positively to the needs of those receiving Shiatsu.

When we describe someone as 'coming from their Hara', we are describing somebody who is well grounded, strongly focused and using the maximum potential of their body and mind together. In the case of a purely physical movement such as sawing a piece of wood, the person

Fig. 2.2: Hara

focused in Hara will use strength from their Hara, by focusing the mind and breath there, so that all the movements necessary to saw the wood will derive from the Hara. In contrast, the person who is not centred in Hara will saw the wood by focusing the breath in the chest and utilize excessive tension and strength from the arms and shoulders.

It is essential that all our movements and techniques in Shiatsu originate from the Hara. Indeed, the proper practice of Shiatsu itself encourages Hara development and centring. Underlying *all* Shiatsu technique is Hara. Diagram 'A' illustrates someone applying pressure with no strength of consciousness in Hara, who is thus forced to use upper body strength. Contrast this with Diagram 'B' which illustrates pressure applied by body weight alone.

For maximum use of Hara it is essential to *keep a low centre of gravity*. This will ensure maximum stability for the giver, and allow the

Fig. 2.3(a): Below Pressure applied with upper body strength

Fig. 2.3(b): Below right Pressure applied with body weight alone neck, shoulders and muscles of the back to relax. When the centre of gravity is too high, the postural muscles must overwork in order to maintain a steady position, resulting in early fatigue.

A low centre of gravity can be maintained by;

- Keeping the knees and hips spread open.
- Keeping the Hara relaxed – to allow natural, deep breathing.
- Directing the mind and breath to Tanden – rather than allowing the concentration of thought to disperse.
- Keeping weight underside – this can be achieved by imagining all the weight of the body accumulating on the undersurfaces. For example, underside of forearms, underside of belly and so on (see Fig. 2.6).

Once a low centre of gravity has been achieved and can be maintained, it is possible for all movements to originate from, and feel connected to, Tanden.

RELAXATION AND COMFORT

If you are tensed up and unable to relax as a giver of Shiatsu, work on it by developing Hara to steady the mind and breath. When you are in actual physical contact with another being, they will consciously or subconsciously know the degree of tension or relaxation in you, because it will be transmitted to them through your touch. Tension and relaxation are infectious. Have you noticed how relaxing it is to have a cat on your lap? Much more so than having a tense and awkward person work on your shoulders! You can only be truly relaxed if you are

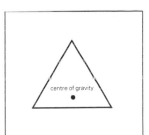

Fig. 2.4: Low centre of gravity (stable)

Fig. 2.5: High centre of gravity (unstable)

Fig. 2.6: Practitioner imagines weight on undersurfaces of body, i.e. palms, lower forearms, lower belly, lower legs, in order to keep a low centre of gravity.

Fig. 2.7: Comfort and ease of position of giver

comfortable, so abandon all dramatic and contorted positions even if they do look impressive, and just get comfortable.

Good Shiatsu can relax someone no matter where they are, but if it can be done in quiet, pleasant, amenable surroundings, so much the better. For both giver and receiver, having an empty stomach without being ravenously hungry, wearing loose cotton rather than statically charged, clingy, artificial materials, avoiding fluorescent lighting and concentrations of electrically-operated devices, will all add to comfort as well as promoting maximum energy levels.

EMPTY MIND

Once steadiness in mind and breath has been achieved, and you are firmly established in Hara, then you can apply Shiatsu with what is known as *Empty Mind*.

Shiatsu is much more about feeling than thinking. If you are constantly thinking what you should be feeling, you will probably feel nothing other than a bag of flesh and bones, and be perplexed as to what to do with it. Also, if you are constantly thinking of what you should be doing, your recipient will be constantly wondering what is going to be done to them. Only by keeping our head 'out of the way', so that our awareness is in our Hara, will we be guided by limitless intuition rather than intellect, which is limited. Thinking is a valid and necessary process in a Shiatsu health assessment, but basic Shiatsu is the natural act of touching and holding another human being, and as such pre-empts thinking. Shiatsu touch does not actually require learning as much as relearning and unlearning poor postural habits and responses. If you have difficulty with this, let a baby or a cat crawl over your back and experience natural basic Shiatsu!

SUPPORT RATHER THAN FORCE

The whole purpose of Shiatsu is to encourage a free flow of energy throughout the body and mind. Where there is tension, there is constriction and consequent restriction of blood and energy circulation. Where there is relaxation, there is 'opening' and consequent free flow of blood and vitality. If we push and poke at our fellow human beings, whether physically or verbally, we meet with resistance as they close up, fight back or withdraw. If we support them they will feel secure, have trust and become receptive to our presence.

The first level of support is therefore to project the idea that you are going to *assist* your recipient rather than impose something upon them.

The second level of support is to ensure stability. The most stable

Leg positions for sidelying

Fig. 2.8(a):

Fig 2.8(b): This variation prevents the recipient from rolling into the prone position

Fig. 2.9: Bodily contact for support in sitting

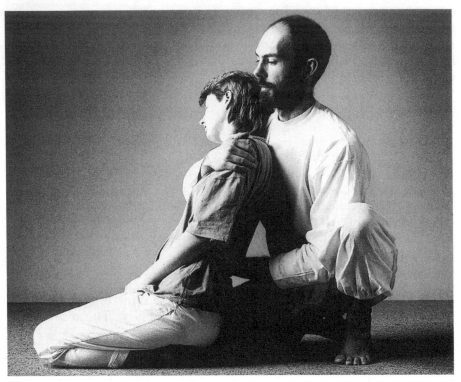

position for the recipient is lying flat in the prone or supine position, whereupon the floor is providing maximum support for the entire body. In this position, no muscular tension is required to offset the effect of gravity upon the posture, unlike in sitting or standing, both of which prohibit total relaxation because the postural muscles remain active.

In sidelying, it is generally beneficial to add support for the head by adding a pillow, and positioning the legs in such a way that prevents a gradual collapsing into prone (see Fig. 2.8).

Basically, the more vertical the recipient's position is for Shiatsu, the more body contact you should give to counteract the force of gravity. Sitting Shiatsu therefore requires maximum body contact to prevent collapse (see Fig. 2.9).

However, total support may not be desirable in every situation. Sometimes you may want to encourage the recipient to 'meet you halfway', especially if you feel they could benefit from gradually taking more responsibility for themselves and be less reliant on others. Part of the art of Shiatsu is to gauge how much support to give. Too much contact and support can be smothering to some people.

The third level of support is the supportive touch. Assuming they are not going to fall over when you apply some of your weight, they may still react defensively if you push or press. By initiating your movement from Hara, and *leaning* rather than pushing, your touch will be welcomed rather than repelled. Consequently the recipient will open up rather than close.

It is the earth which ultimately supports everything in our life, and the closest we can get to the earth is to lie flat on the ground. This is one reason why Shiatsu is better done on the floor rather than on a table. Also, the more grounded we are as givers of Shiatsu, the more support we can give. Once more, good Hara is the key.

Finally, the fourth level of support is to be accessible if the receiver needs to clarify any after-effects arising out of a Shiatsu session, in which case a supportive word from you at the right time will put their mind at ease.

POSITIVE CONNECTION

Connection is really an extension of support. You cannot support somebody unless you are in some way connected to them, yet you can connect with somebody in such a way as to undermine their support; for example, by physically pushing them over, or by making some verbal connection that undermines their confidence, trust and optimism. Consequently, connection can be positive or negative, and as givers of Shiatsu we have the opportunity to enhance positive connection.

Positive connection has both a physical and psychological aspect, which together form the strongest possible energetic connection. The first opportunity to be positively connected is to be open and friendly and to deliberately seek some area of common ground between yourself and the recipient. This should be aimed for as soon as you meet or speak to the recipient, although it will probably be achieved already with those recipients who are family or friends.

On the physical level, the touch of one finger or thumb on a remote part of the body, compared to simultaneous touch from two hands, is very different. When two hands consciously contact the recipient a circuit is completed giving a sense of unification between the giver and receiver, and between the two hands in contact. Touching with only one hand however, is much more likely to result in a feeling of intrusion, or at best localized soothing.

What works best, with a few exceptions, is to have both hands in contact with the person, but kept slightly apart, rather than one on top of the other. The giver should then focus on Hara rather than on hands or thumbs. This will result in the receiver experiencing the two contact places as if they were one large single area of contact. If sustained longer, the receiver will experience the sensation of a single unified contact deep within their being. Meanwhile, the giver will experience this as a distinct current of energy or 'echo' between the two hands. This may feel like a circle of continuity through and with the receiver, between the hands and through one's own Hara. A truly experienced practitioner can maintain this sensation when one hand is stationary and the other is moving, which greatly enhances the quality of continuity, as discussed later.

PERPENDICULAR PRESSURE

Since Shiatsu is concerned with harmonizing Ki, it is important that pressure, whether applied with palms, fingers, thumbs or whatever, is applied at right angles to the surface of the body. This is because the surface distortion caused by non-perpendicular pressure tends to compress and stretch the tissues unevenly around the point of contact. This is very good for increasing blood circulation and lymphatic drainage, but does not have sufficient energetic penetration to make a direct connection with the Ki within the Channels. Instead it may encourage its random dispersal. If a person is very weak and deficient in Ki, this method could upset the delicate interplay of Ki still further, and cause the recipient to become even more deficient. Although rubbing and shaking techniques can be useful as a general warm up for the muscles and a 'loosener' for the joints, one should generally avoid overdoing this with the weak, chronically Ki-deficient person.

Perpendicular pressure produces a 'centring' quality by creating a steady, even epicentre of contact, which has a magnetic attraction to Ki, and is therefore very tonifying for that area if held for several seconds.

Perpendicular penetration is even more crucial when connecting directly with a Tsubo. Since a Tsubo is shaped like a vase, non-perpendicular contact will fail to get beyond its neck, and therefore make little or no contact with Channel Ki, unless the Tsubo is Jitsu, and Ki is blocked in the neck of that Tsubo.

For the receiver, the feeling of incorrectly angled contact will be like superficial manipulation of the surface of the body, which after a short time can become tedious. Off-centre, deep physical pressure can feel very irritating, painful and invasive. Deep connection is determined purely by focus, angle and awareness centred in Hara, and has nothing to do with how hard the Tsubo is physically pressed. In fact, too much physical pressure merely causes defensive reactions which block Ki connection.

Practise accurate perpendicular connection with Tsubos. It is not difficult to master with a little time and patience. Without some sensitivity in this area, the effect of your Shiatsu will be severely impaired.

Fig. 2.10: Dispersal quality of non-perpendicular pressure, compared to 'magnetic' tonifying quality of perpendicular pressure

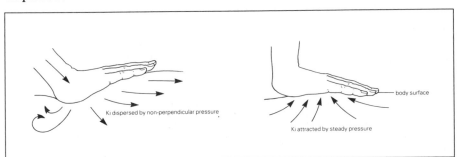

Ki dispersed by non-perpendicular pressure

body surface

Ki attracted by steady pressure

STATIONARY PRESSURE

Because the deepest Shiatsu treatment is the tonification of the deficient Kyo Tsubos, it is essential to understand that stationary pressure will be used more frequently than variable pressure techniques. Stationary pressure is deeply penetrating and therefore able to connect with deficient Ki which lies more deeply below the surface than excess Ki. Also, sustained pressure calms the internal organs by stimulating the parasympathetic nervous system. Two to ten seconds of pressure generally suffices, although up to forty-five seconds is sometimes required. In general, stationary perpendicular pressure is the main method of tonifying the Kyo, whereas non-perpendicular techniques such as shaking, circling, rocking, kneading, or anything which involves more movement will sedate or disperse Jitsu. Remember however, that *no* lasting sedation of Jitsu will be achieved unless the Kyo that caused it has been tonified. Various techniques are described in Chapter 3.

Fig. 2.11: Non-perpendicular pressure may connect with a Tsubo full of energy, but fail to make any connection with one that is more empty

TECHNICAL ABILITY

To give Shiatsu you must have a repertoire of techniques to draw upon. If you are a beginner you will find it easier to stick to a regular sequence of techniques. With more experience you will gain the confidence to select appropriate techniques to suit the recipient's unique energetic imbalances and eventually be able to create or adapt techniques to fit any given circumstance. All that is required is constant diligent practice.

Actually, your skill as a practitioner is not a reflection of how many techniques you know, but of your proficiency in delivering them well. It is best to learn a few fundamental techniques for the face up, face down, side lying and sitting positions. Experience will automatically present more advanced variations if all the principles of Shiatsu described in this chapter are integrated into your work. Quality rather than quantity is the key.

Fig. 2.12: Pressure on the neck of a deficient Tsubo may create distortions detrimental to Ki flow

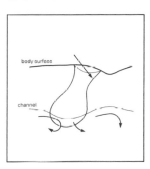

Avoid the egocentricity of 'performing' Shiatsu. It is possible to look very gymnastic and dextrous with your technique, but if that is your reason for doing it, the therapeutic value of your session will be severely diminished. This is because the more you are concerned with how you look and rate in the eyes of the recipient, the less you will be able to focus upon them. Consequently, the less you will be able to help them, because sensitivity to Ki gathers where your consciousness is directed. For this reason empathy and Ki sensitivity are inversely proportional to egocentricity.

CONTINUITY

To receive good Shiatsu is to experience a feeling of integration throughout the body and between the body and mind. This only happens however, if there is a sense of connection, support and continuity from the giver. A session should therefore be conducted in a co-ordinated flowing manner rather than as a disjointed amalgam of random techniques. Each technique should be a logical extension of the previous one, and wherever possible, contact should be maintained as the hand moves from one area to the next. For example, if the thumb is applied to area A, then B, then C, the hand should glide over the surface between A, B and C, rather than taking it away from the body each time (see Fig. 2.13). Making and breaking contact continuously will inhibit the receiver's ability to relax to deeper levels, because they will be unsure where the contact will be felt next, or perhaps they will try to anticipate your movements upon them. What we want is for them to experience the 'now' because of the reality of contact is only in the present.

Just consider, if you the giver do not know where you are going or why, the receiver is hardly going to be overwhelmed with confidence in you (see Fig. 2.14).

CHANNEL CONTINUITY

Shiatsu not only makes use of the fixed acupuncture points, but also uses those transient Tsubos which manifest elsewhere along a Channel. Consequently, it is possible to work on an entire Channel rather than on the classical acupoints alone. By keeping a support hand stationary, and

Fig. 2.13: Hand glides over body area between points of pressure

the other hand working along the course of a Channel, we begin to feel points which react to our presence, either directly in the moving hand, indirectly in the support hand, or in both hands. By feeling reactions between both the support and moving hands, we begin to experience the energetic quality of the Channel, therefore enabling us to follow its course via the Tsubos that appear within it, tonifying, dispersing or calming them as required. This is known as 'Channel Continuity' because the pattern of where and when the body is touched is based upon sensitivity and connection to the Channel's flow throughout its whole length, or sections of its length, rather than solely upon the actions of individual classical points.

FLUENCY

Fluency means being well practised in a wide variety of techniques. It is the ability to give a full body Shiatsu, or a specific treatment without having to think about technique. When a language is spoken fluently, one does not have to search so hard for words to express what one wants to say. Likewise, when a Shiatsu practitioner wants to produce a particular effect, the techniques should manifest of themselves.

Fluency is only possible through repeated practice. For the beginner it is best to practise set technique sequences so that the need to decide what to do next is eliminated. This will leave more space for developing touch qualities.

For the giver of Shiatsu, fluency frees the mind to remain in the 'now', which is the only time and place where the receiver's level of vitality can be perceived through touch. The 'now' is missed if the mind

Fig. 2.14: Making and breaking contact leaves the recipient anticipating or bewildered as to where you will touch next

is locked in the past trying to remember relevant techniques to suit the occasion.

Another important aspect of Shiatsu fluency is the ability to move from one part of the body to another with minimal effort and disturbance, especially where it involves moving from one side of the recipient to the other. This is known as *transitioning*.

A good transition is when the giver has moved without the receiver noticing. Many Shiatsu sessions have compromised their relaxing benefits because the giver has fumbled about changing positions without having given due consideration to this aspect of their practice.

EMPATHY

Empathy is the ability and inclination to appreciate how another person is feeling. The strongest form of empathy is in the ability to actually 'feel' how another person is feeling. The two ingredients which enhance empathy are focus in Hara and genuine concern for the other's well-being. Really, these two ingredients need to be united for full effect. Genuine concern is reflected in the level of openness in your heart. This openness, when anchored to a grounded sense of Hara, enables the giver to put him or herself in the position of the receiver and sympathize with

Fig. 2.15: Interplay of personal Ki with universal Ki

them. If heart only is involved, the giver could easily become thrown off-centre by over-sympathizing with any strong emotions exhibited by the recipient. The grounding from Hara however, will give a degree of objectivity and consequent clarity.

What happens if you give Shiatsu with strong Hara but a closed heart is that you may pick up the general level of vitality, but have no sense of their emotional needs. Without the element of compassion, there could also be an inclination towards heavy-handed techniques which could produce unnecessary physical pain.

If the heart is open, but the Hara is closed, the giver will use too much energy through inefficient application of body weight. More significantly, the giver will give too much of his or herself emotionally and energetically without harvesting the limitless universal Ki which can be channelled through one's body by connecting heart to Hara. Fig. 2.15 illustrates the interplay of personal Ki with universal Ki.

Chapter 3

The Tools of Shiatsu

No special equipment is required to give Shiatsu. All you need is your body, plus enough clean floor space for the recipient to lie down, and for you to move around them. The floor should be comfortable but firm. A futon one or two layers thick is ideal, although a thick carpet covered with a sheet will suffice. A thin cotton or silk cloth approximately 18″ square is useful for applying techniques to the neck and face, because Shiatsu feels better and is less obtrusive through a barrier of thin natural fibres. Technique applied to bare skin tends to be more superficial because the sensation of skin contact distracts from feeling the deeper and more subtle presence of Ki. The superficial sensory nerve endings are most prolific on the surface, so a cloth barrier will dampen down the surface tactile sensations and allow the receiver to feel the deeper connection.

For this reason it is essential that the receiver is completely covered in a single layer of clothing throughout the session. This has the added advantage of making sexual innuendo and embarrassment less likely to manifest. Also it means that Shiatsu can be given almost anywhere. Even in the office, Shiatsu to the head, neck and shoulders can be applied.

It might seem from first impressions that a Tsubo would be easier to find and feel on bare skin, but a little practice through thin cloth reveals this to be untrue.

GENERAL PRINCIPLES OF TONIFYING, DISPERSING, AND CALMING KI

Tonifying   To tonify Ki, apply stationary pressure with a thumb or fingertip perpendicular to the mouth of the Tsubo, so that a deep connection can be made. Hold the pressure until you feel some reaction there. Sometimes it feels like the vase shaped Tsubo is filling up with Ki. This should take from about ten seconds to four minutes. If you feel nothing after four minutes, move on to another Tsubo, perhaps returning later to the ones which are slow to react.

It is important that the pressure is not too deep as this could have the counterproductive effect of dispersing Ki, as well as feeling invasive and painful to the recipient. You should go into the Tsubo with the attitude of *meeting* the Ki. Remember that Ki goes where the mind is focused. Therefore, you can be more effective with less pressure if you clearly *visualize* the area lying slightly deep to your finger's depth of penetration. In this way, the recipient's Ki will be drawn to meet your Ki, which will be projected slightly ahead of your fingertip. If and when a connection is felt, reduce the pressure slightly to allow Ki to fill the Tsubo.

This principle of 'Ki attraction' can be compared to touching the surface of water with the tip of your finger. The surface tension of water allows itself to be drawn up by your fingertips, so that as you slowly pull your finger away, the water follows. However, unlike water, a new level of Ki will persist in the Tsubo even after the finger has been removed. That is why the more sensitive and focused the practitioner becomes, the less pressure need be applied. Consequently, a recipient in the hands of an experienced practitioner will experience a deep connection from a relatively light touch.

With practice, sensitivity and a great deal of focus, broad tonification of an area can also be achieved with palms, elbows, knees or feet.

Dispersing

As we have indicated, it is possible to disperse (or sedate) Ki by deeply penetrating a Jitsu Tsubo. However, this is invasive and painful and can be likened to dispersing a crowd with a baton charge; dispersal is achieved but nobody is very happy as a result.

The reason for using a dispersal technique is to unblock a concentration of Ki so that it can move smoothly along the Channel. To achieve this, you can ease your thumb or finger a little way into the Tsubo, and apply a rotatory movement, imagining the Ki being loosened and dispersed. Then, progressively ease the pressure, so that you spiral out of the point. Alternatively, 'pumping' in and out of a mildly Jitsu Tsubo is sometimes effective.

It is worth remembering that a firm support hand on a nearby Kyo area will usually speed up dispersal from the Jitsu region, as well as minimize pain. However, if an area is very full, these dispersal techniques can create too much pain. Extremely full areas are best left alone, because if you develop enough skill in finding and tonifying Kyo areas, the Jitsu areas will often react by dispersing spontaneously.

Stretching, squeezing and shaking techniques all effectively disperse areas which are generally Jitsu.

Calming

Calming is a gentler type of dispersal. Sometimes an area of the body, or a Tsubo, presents a Jitsu quality because the Ki in that area is hyperactive, rather than too concentrated. In this situation, a calming technique is indicated. Calming is achieved by simply covering the area with your palms and remaining calm and peaceful yourself. Do exactly what you would do if you were trying to calm an anxious or upset friend; keep centred and apply a supportive touch.

It sometimes happens that a very hysterical person is calmed with a slap. Slapping a 'hysterical' area of the body (not the head) also works in Shiatsu, but you must be **very** experienced and confident in your abilities to try this technique. A gentle stroking action along a Channel is also very calming. However, remember that nothing you do will be calming if you, the practitioner are not calm and centred yourself.

The parts of the body which can be used to apply technique are:

- Palms
- Thumbs
- Fingers
- Elbows
- Knees
- Feet

PALMS

Although less specific than the fingertips or thumbs, the palms are more soothing, with less potential for causing pain or damage. The whole surface area of the palm should be kept in full contact with the recipient so that the hand can mould around the contours of the body. The palms will therefore lie more flat on the back, or curl to envelop an arm or an ankle. The palms and fingers must remain relaxed (see Fig. 3.1).

Arms should remain outstretched, but with the elbows unlocked. The angle of the body in relation to the arms will determine the amount of pressure applied (see Fig. 3.2).

When closer body contact is preferred, it is sometimes useful to have the arms angled 90° at the elbow, with the knee or inner thigh

Fig. 3.1: Palms and fingers relaxed

Fig. 3.2: Angle of body in relation to arms

supporting your upper arm. There is however a slight reduction in the connection of Ki flow between Hara and palms with this method (see Fig. 3.3).

Keeping both hands in contact but spread apart is the most therapeutic method because of the increased connection and support. This method enables one hand to 'listen' while the other hand is active, or allows one to tonify while the other calms or disperses.

Support Hand Technique

Fig. 3.3: Arms angled 90° at elbow

Fig. 3.4: Support hand technique: tonifying hand should be applied at right angles

support hand

tonifying hand

Fig. 3.5: Hands lying one on top of the other

Palm Overlap Technique Hands lying one on top of the other can be used when a malleable 'wave like' action is required.

Circular Rotations/Shaking Although more superficial in effect than focused, stationary, perpendicular pressure, rotations and shaking are especially effective for relieving muscular tensions around the shoulder blades, or for stimulating warmth in the pelvic region when applied to the sacrum. Note that the connective tissues should be moved over the underlying bone rather than merely frictioning the surface.

Grasping This method is especially useful when applied to the arms and legs. One

Fig. 3.6: Circular rotations on shoulder blades

Fig. 3.7: One hand clasps limb for support, other moves along limb

hand clasps the limb for support, while the other moves along the limb. A firm support hand is very important.

With fingers interlocked, pressure is applied simultaneously with the heels of both hands. This method is used to squeeze the muscles either side of the lumbar spine, from the kidney region down to the pelvis (see Fig. 3.8).

Double Palm Squeezing

Holding the palms one to six inches away from the body has a warming and tonifying effect if the giver is relaxed with their awareness centred in Tanden. This method is especially effective when applied over the face,

Off the Body Method

which can be a nice way to conclude a session. When Ki sensitivity is developed, local excess or deficiency of Ki can be clearly assessed using this technique.

Fig. 3.8: Fingers interlocked, pressure applied with heels of both hands

Fig. 3.9: Palms off the body

THUMBS

The thumb is a very widely used tool for Shiatsu. It is shorter and thicker than the fingers, with only one interphalangeal joint instead of two, making it the strongest individual digit. Strong pressure can therefore be applied and sustained where necessary.

Fig. 3.10: Using ball of thumb

The ball of the thumb is used for most applications, although the area near the tip can be used when working with light pressure between small muscle groups such as in the neck.

People with stiff interphalangeal joints tend to emphasize the tip too much and are advised to adjust this, as it can be painful for the receiver. Some people have very flexible interphalangeal joints, and run the risk of overstraining them. If your thumb is of this type (see Fig. 3.12) you should use the digital ball and not the joint; and are advised to make more use of the other tools such as the palms or multiple fingers.

Fig. 3.11: Using area near tip

For stability it is preferable to place the other four digits lightly on the body. In an area of acute Ki distortion this allows the four fingers to remain stationary and to tonify, while the thumb actively disperses (see Fig. 3.13).

Open Hand Method

Alternatively, the four remaining digits can be formed into a fist so that the index finger can support the thumb (see Fig. 3.14). The latter is particularly useful for those with hypermobile interphalangeal joints.

Closed Hand Method

Fig. 3.12: Overstraining of interphalangeal joint

Fig. 3.13: Four fingers stationary and tonifying, thumb disperses

Fig. 3.14: Fist method

Figs 3.15(a) and (b) show other variations of thumb application which enable greater pressure to be applied to a Tsubo. However, such heavy pressure is unnecessary if treatment is accurately focused on the Kyo areas.

FINGERS

Fig. 3.15(a) Below: Thumb adjacent

Fig. 3.15(b) Below right: Thumb overlap

The fingertips are excellent tools for sensing the quality of Channel Ki because of their rich supply of sensory nerve endings. Thumbnails and fingernails should be kept short.

Fig. 3.16: Three fingers for Hara energy assessment

Using the second, third and fourth fingers simultaneously (i.e. the middle three) is the most versatile method. The fingers can be together or slightly apart. The thumb should be relaxed and the fingers strong (constant use of this method will quickly strengthen them). Like all Shiatsu techniques, the movement must originate from Hara, with a sense of connection to Tanden. This will give a sense of strength coming through the elbows rather than fatigue and tension accumulating in the wrist (see Fig. 3.16).

This method is used for Hara energy assessment, tracking the Channel Ki flow, and for finely tuned Ki projection and penetration.

Three Finger Method

This can be used in the same way as three fingers. A wider space between

Four Finger Method

Fig. 3.17: Dispersing tension in intercostal muscles

Fig. 3.18: Pressure to side of nose

the fingers produces a configuration excellent for dispersing tension in the intercostal muscles between the ribs.

Index Finger Method Place your middle finger on top of your index finger to give it extra support. This is a useful alternative for those with hypermobile interphalangeal thumb joints. It is very good for applying pressure to the side of the nose (see Fig. 3.18).

Fig. 3.19: Kenbiki

Fig. 3.20: Pummelling

SUBSIDIARY HAND TECHNIQUES

The subsidiary hand techniques are occasionally used to disperse and calm Jitsu areas, as well as increase circulation of blood and lymph to the skin and superficial muscles. These techniques should not be applied to chronically weakened clients who have insufficient Ki, and therefore need stationary pressure to tonify their Kyo rather than dispersal techniques. (See Figs 3.19–3.25.)

Fig. 3.21: Loose finger chopping

Fig. 3.22: Right Cupping

Fig. 3.23: Far right Double hand cushioning

Fig. 3.24: Rocking (very gently is OK for Kyo recipients; more vigorous is more dispersing)

Claw Technique Thumb and fingers are slightly curled to form a claw. The claw is then pressed into the body and quickly withdrawn as if imagining strands being pulled out of the body. In reality excess Ki is being pulled out of the area being worked on. This technique is used to disperse pockets of accumulated Ki (Jitsu areas) or stagnant Ki around the shoulder blades and buttocks, by removing it from the body completely. It is not used on the weaker client, or on Kyo areas. (See Fig. 3.26.)

Fig. 3.25: Knuckle rolling (on the feet)

Fig. 3.26: Ki being pulled out of the body

The middle and index fingers are pressed simultaneously either side of the spinal column in small infants, or in the intercostal spaces close to either side of the sternum in adults.

'Vee' Finger Technique

The thumb and index finger are spread wide. Pressure is applied through the wide angle 'vee' shape, with pressure falling mainly on the

'Dragon's Mouth' Technique

Fig. 3.27: Dragon's Mouth to occiput

Fig. 3.28: Dragon's Mouth with both hands to waistline

proximal joint of the index finger. The 'Dragon's mouth' can be used to apply pressure just above the knee or to the occiput. Both hands can be placed together to apply pressure to the waist in the sidelying position (see Figs 3.27, 3.28).

Fig. 3.29: Variety of elbow joint angles

ELBOWS

The elbows, or the area of forearm close to the elbows, can be used to apply strong pressure to the back, hips and feet. They should be used with care, and applied only to areas which have already been palpated by the hands. This is because they are far less sensitive than the hands.

An acutely flexed elbow joint gives the strongest pressure, which in most cases is too much. A more open elbow joint gives a more comfortable pressure, which can be varied according to the angle of the elbow joint. It is essential to keep the wrist relaxed and fist open. (See Fig. 3.29.)

The elbow should not be used before a high level of sensitivity has developed in the hands. Premature use of elbow techniques will reduce the number of friends willing to receive your Shiatsu!

KNEES

The knees can give very firm pressure, so should be used with discretion only to areas previously checked by the hands. They can be applied individually or both together, but the majority of your body weight should be kept back on your haunches, or equally distributed through the hands.

Maximum support should be given so that the knees can be instantly removed if necessary to ensure the receiver's comfort and your own stability. (See Fig. 3.30.)

FEET

Feet can be used as a tool for Shiatsu, and although they are less sensitive than the hands, they can give a very 'earthy' ingredient to a

Fig 3.30: Knees on inner thighs in sidelying

session. This is perhaps because they spend most of their time in contact with the ground. If you intend to use your feet you should walk around in bare feet as much as possible to give them an even greater earthy quality.

Using the feet gives you a chance to stand up if you have been giving Shiatsu with your hands for several hours. They can be used to tonify the ankles, which in turn helps to tonify the kidneys (see Fig 3.31). Generally however, they are more useful for temporarily dispersing Jitsu areas in the limbs by using a rapid shaking technique, but with light pressure (see Fig 3.32). This may be useful for dispersing excessive

Fig. 3.31: Standing on ankles to tonify the kidneys . . . but only if ankles are flexible enough

Fig. 3.32: Vigorous shaking of foot on calf muscles – *avoid knee joint*

surface tension when it is masking underlying Kyo, thus rendering the Kyo more accessible to hand palpation.

Feet are useful tools to anchor the recipient's body when certain stretches are applied (see Fig. 3.33).

Fig. 3.33: Body anchored in prone lying, leg stretched

To apply Shiatsu using the feet requires that you keep your centre of gravity as low as possible by constantly imagining the feet are being filled from Tanden with sand or some other heavy substance.

BREATHING

The correct way to breathe for both the giver and receiver comes automatically provided both are relaxed. The level of relaxation in the receiver is largely influenced by the degree of relaxation in the giver, due to the close proximity and energy-based nature of Shiatsu.

When pressure or stretch is applied, it is natural for both giver and receiver to gently exhale. Inhalation naturally takes place when pressure is released. The more relaxed you are, the longer will be the period of no-breathing between exhalation and inhalation. The no-breathing phase is when there is maximum receptivity to subtle changes in muscle tone or Ki flow. However, it is quite common to discover that your recipient simply cannot fully relax because they are not in touch with their breathing. For these people it is helpful to tell them to consciously breathe out as you apply pressure. After several repetitions of dictated

Fig. 3.34:
Mechanically assisting exhalation using palm pressure on the ribs, in supine

breathing, they usually make the correction and all is well. In some cases it is helpful to apply pressure to their lower ribs as you tell them to exhale, thus giving their lungs some mechanical assistance (see Fig 3.34).

Chapter 4

Shiatsu Channel Outlines

Some styles of Shiatsu use no Channels at all, some use the traditional acupuncture Channels, while others use the extended Channel system expounded by Shizuto Masunaga. For family orientated Shiatsu it is not necessary to use the Channels to achieve basic relaxation and to alleviate minor aches and pains. However, even with family orientated Shiatsu, one begins to feel specific differences between different areas within a given space, such as say, the thigh. If Ki sensitivity is consciously being developed through the diligent practice of Shiatsu – and perhaps reinforced through Aikido or Qi Gong – and if the mind of the exponent is curious enough, the Channels begin to present themselves. Having said that, it would take a long time to recognize them spontaneously for what they are, and what they represent. Hence we give you a map.

The Classical Channels present a grid for the location and treatment of fixed Tsubos. However, tactile experience reveals that each Channel can be strongly influenced by Shiatsu applied to certain other areas of the body. These areas or 'extensions' are most clearly represented in the limbs. Each of the six Classical Channels in the arms have corresponding energy extensions in the legs. Likewise, the six leg Channels have related extensions in the arms. These extensions sometimes follow the course of another Channel. For example, the Heart Channel's extension at the postero-medial aspect of the thigh lies over the Classical Kidney Channel.

Since no fixed Tsubos appear on the extensions, they are of little value to acupuncturists. However, since the Channels are affected by the penetration of touch into the extensions, they prove invaluable to the Shiatsu therapist.

This idea of Channel extension was first put forward by Shizuto Masunaga, who was primarily responsible for promoting their use.

Both the Classical Channels and their extended Channel pathways are presented as a map on the following pages.

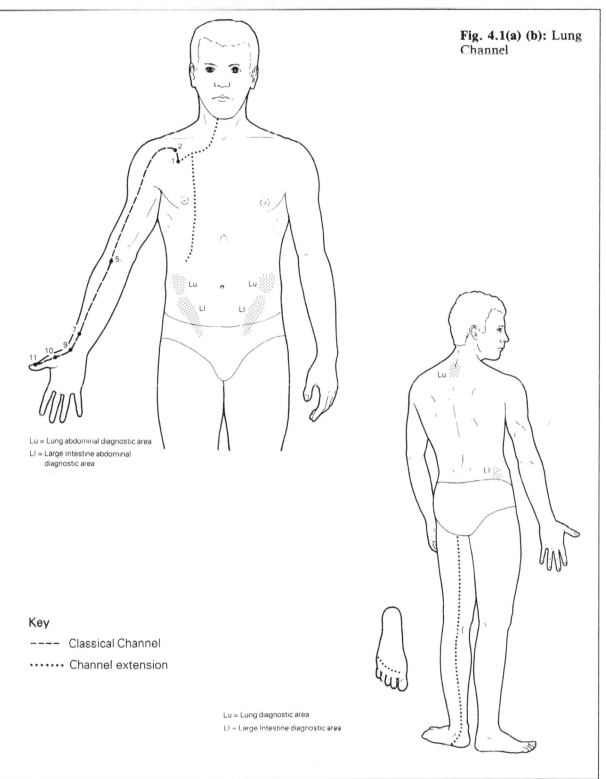

Fig. 4.1(a) (b): Lung Channel

Lu = Lung abdominal diagnostic area
LI = Large Intestine abdominal diagnostic area

Key

---- Classical Channel

······ Channel extension

Lu = Lung diagnostic area
LI = Large Intestine diagnostic area

Fig. 4.2(a) (b): Large Intestine Channel

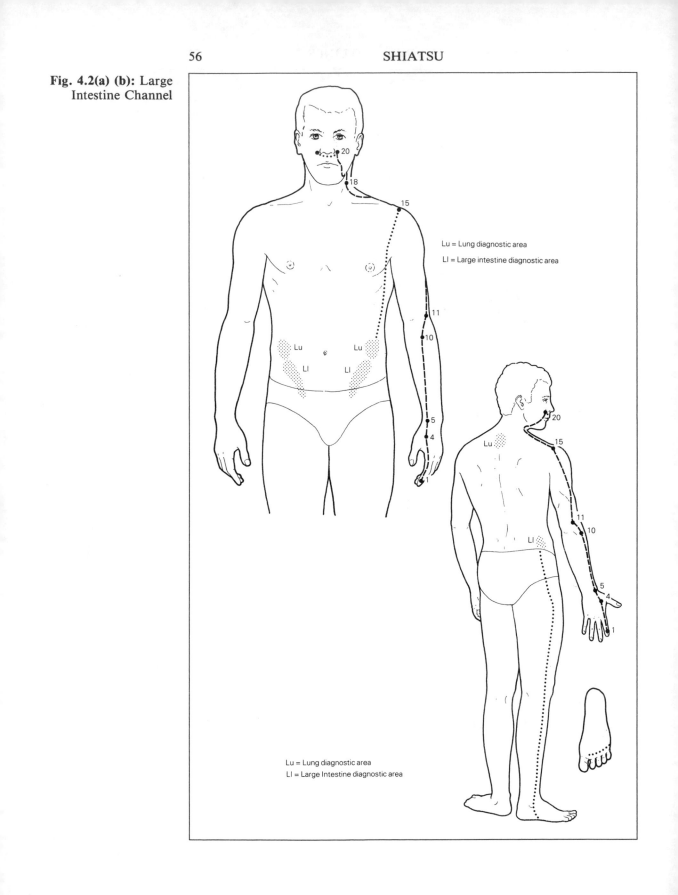

Lu = Lung diagnostic area

LI = Large intestine diagnostic area

Lu = Lung diagnostic area

LI = Large Intestine diagnostic area

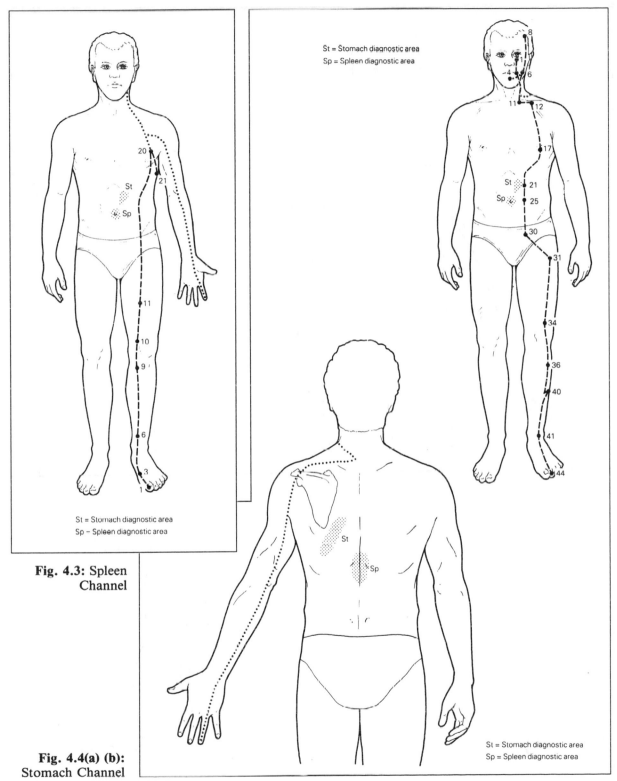

St = Stomach diagnostic area
Sp = Spleen diagnostic area

Fig. 4.3: Spleen Channel

Fig. 4.4(a) (b): Stomach Channel

Ht = Heart diagnostic area
SI = Small Intestine diagnostic area

Fig. 4.5(a) (b): Heart
Channel

Fig. 4.6(a) (b): Small Intestine Channel

SI = Small Intestine diagnostic area

Ht = Heart diagnostic area
SI = Small Intestine diagnostic area

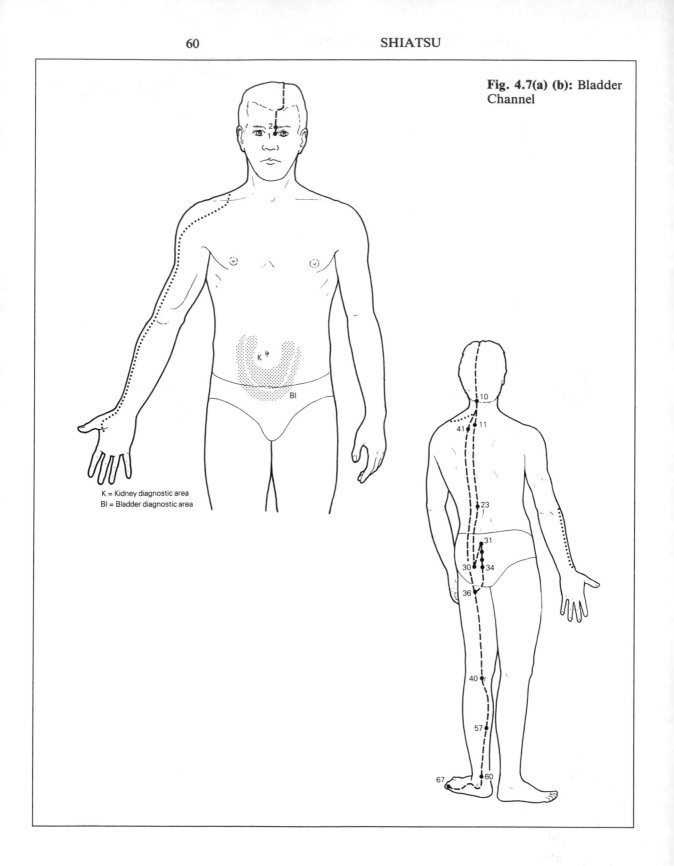

Fig. 4.7(a) (b): Bladder Channel

K = Kidney diagnostic area
Bl = Bladder diagnostic area

K = Kidney diagnostic area
Bl = Bladder diagnostic area

K = Kidney diagnostic area
Bl = Bladder diagnostic area

Fig. 4.8(a) (b): Kidney
Channel

HP = Heart Protector diagnostic area
TH = Triple Heater diagnostic area

HP   TH

Fig. 4.9(a) (b): Heart
Protector Channel

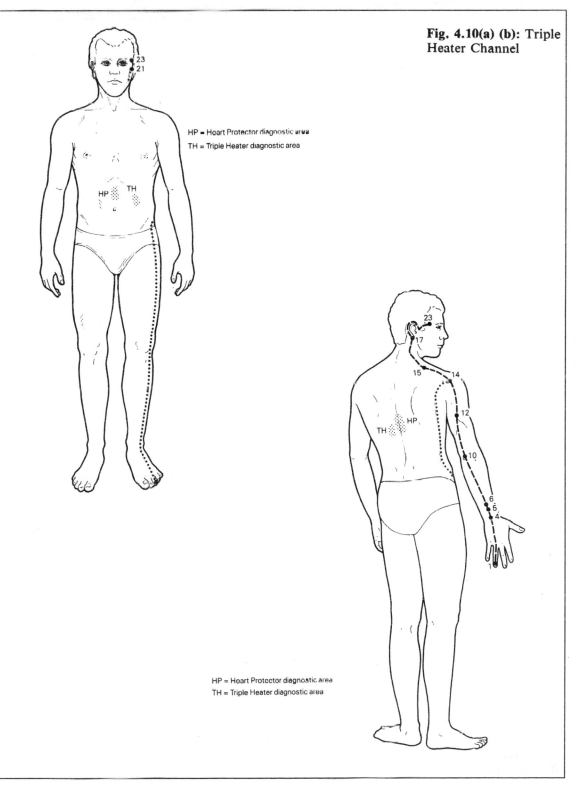

Fig. 4.10(a) (b): Triple Heater Channel

HP = Heart Protector diagnostic area
TH = Triple Heater diagnostic area

HP = Heart Protector diagnostic area
TH = Triple Heater diagnostic area

GB = Gall Bladder diagnostic area
Li = Liver diagnostic area

Fig. 4.11: Liver Channel

GB = Gall Bladder diagnostic area
Li = Liver diagnostic area

Fig. 4.12(a) (b): Gall Bladder Channel

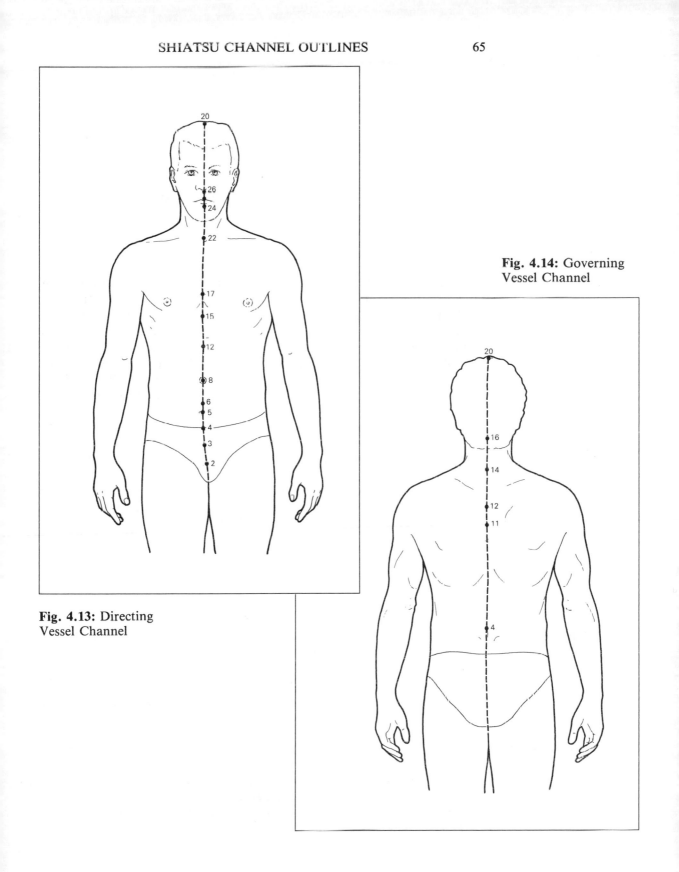

Fig. 4.14: Governing Vessel Channel

Fig. 4.13: Directing Vessel Channel

Chapter 5

Basic Shiatsu Technique

This chapter will present a variety of techniques for each main position in which the receiver can be placed, namely, face down, face up, sidelying and sitting, giving an overall general sequence which is by no means exhaustive, as the possibilities for technique variation are endless. You should bear in mind that each of us are of unique physical proportions so that all of these techniques will suit some people, and some techniques will suit all people. Most of us however, will be inclined to abandon certain techniques and make slight adaptations to others. This adds to the creativity of Shiatsu, which is important if a flexible reaction to the infinite variety of interrelationships between giver and receiver is to be maintained. Please adapt, adjust and accommodate without sacrificing any of the essential elements of Shiatsu outlined in Chapter 2.

If you are the type of person who prefers to work with a well defined structure, then these sequences can provide a basic framework into which you can add the stretches described in Chapter 6.

FACE DOWN POSITION

1. Baby Walking   This technique is so named because the giver should simply walk over the receiver's back and buttocks using the palms, with the same lack of tension and natural use of body weight as a baby would do. Keep the palms relaxed and avoid the spinal column. This technique is comforting for the receiver and helps the giver 'connect' (see Fig. 5.1).

2. Palming   This is similar to baby walking except you keep one hand stationary while the other hand explores the back. Consciousness should be in the stationary hand to feel for any changes in muscle tone or movement of Ki, and to maintain a sense of connection between the two hands. This technique is more effective if the support hand is connected to a particularly Kyo area.

One hand on the scapula, the other hand on the buttocks. Repeat crossing arms and also try using forearms instead of hands (see Fig. 5.2).

3. Diagonal Stretch

Rock from your Hara rather than just from your hands. Find the receiver's natural rocking rhythm and go with it. Gently is very calming; more vigorous is dispersing (see Fig. 5.3).

4. Rocking

Move the skin and connective tissues over the sacral bone rather than friction rub the surface. This technique stimulates circulation to the pelvic region and can move Ki that has stagnated there, but should be avoided if the Bladder Channel is Kyo (see Fig. 5.4).

5. Sacral Rub

Fig. 5.1: Baby walking: relaxed body; weight underside; maximum connection

Fig. 5.2: Diagonal stretch

Fig. 5.3: Rocking

Fig. 5.4: Sacral rub

Fig. 5.5: Retreating cat

Walking hands from buttocks to shoulders and down arms. This will prepare Bladder Channel for subsequent thumb pressure technique (see Fig. 5.5).

6. 'Retreating Cat'

7. Thumb Down Bladder Channel

Fig. 5.6(a): Above
Thumb down Bladder Channel – 2 thumb technique

Fig. 5.6(b): Left
Thumb down Bladder Channel – 1 thumb technique with support hand

8. Working on Bladder Channel in Legs

Fig. 5.7: Working on Bladder Channel in legs. First use palms, then use thumbs

Fig. 5.8: Forearm into sole of foot

9. Forearms into Sole of Foot

Support hand clasps firmly around ankle, to tonify Kidney and Bladder Channels. Make sure their instep is fully supported by your thigh. This may be uncomfortable for you until you have developed sufficient flexibility in toe and ankle plantarflexion. (See Fig. 5.8.)

FACE UP POSITION

1. Pulling Heels

Hold heels rather than grasp ankles. Rest forearms on thighs and lean back. The feeling should be of lengthening through the chest into the

Fig. 5.9: Pulling heels

Fig. 5.10(a): Below left
Knee to chest

back of the head. Shaking from side to side with a gentle 'whip-like'
action is also useful from this position as a general loosener.

Fig. 5.10(b): Below
Knee to chest

Two variations illustrated (Fig. 5.10 a and b). This technique mildly
lengthens the lumbar and gluteal musculature.

2. Knee to Chest

It is very supportive to keep your body in full contact with the
recipient's leg (see Fig. 5.11).

3. Hip Rotations

Hold their foot 'protectively' into your Hara and gently rotate your
whole body. This is incredibly supportive, nurturing and 'grounding'
for the receiver and one of the most centring and relaxing techniques to
give. The other leg can be worked on in the same way.

4. Baby-Rocking the Foot

Fig. 5.11: Hip rotation

Fig. 5.12: Baby-rocking the foot

5. Hand to Hara This is a comforting way to relax the receiver while tonifying the Heart Channel. It is very centring to give. Use palm first, then thumb on upper arm, fingertips on forearm (see Fig. 5.13).

Finger Tip Occiput Support This is excellent for tonifying the Gall Bladder Channel if it is Kyo in the occipital area. Fingertips are contacting GB20 and can connect with all

Fig. 5.13: Hand to Hara

the occipital points (BL 10 and GV 16). Avoid working directly on the occiput if this area is Jitsu, because it could bring on a headache.

Fig. 5.14: Finger tip occiput support

SIDELYING POSITION

Rotate the shoulder with receiver's forearm resting over yours, keeping maximum body contact and moving your whole body from your Hara. This enables the recipient to relax into it better (see Fig. 5.15).

1. Shoulder Girdle Rotation

Forearm connects to front of shoulder. Lean weight through both hands simultaneously (see Fig. 5.16).

2. Head Press

Fig. 5.15: Shoulder girdle rotation

Fig. 5.16: Head press

Support hand rests diagonally opposite occiput, near forehead. Forearms connect to front of shoulder. Thumbs or fingertips connect into occipital Tsubos including GB 20, BL 10 and GV 16, and then into neck from occiput to nape of neck (see Fig. 5.17).

3. Occipital Opening/Neck Release

Use fingertips or heel of hand to disperse Jitsu in Small Intestine, Gall Bladder or Triple Heater Channels in the scapula area (see Fig. 5.18).

4. Shoulder Girdle Dispersing Technique

Fig. 5.17: Occipital opening/neck release

Fig. 5.18: Shoulder girdle dispersing technique

5. Scapula Loosening Scapula is folded over fingertips. Working hand is supported by the thigh. Difficulty getting under one side only can indicate postural imbalance such as scoliosis. Right scapula stiffness may indicate a congested liver. Left scapula stiffness may indicate acid Stomach. Stiffness in both may be due to Liver congestion; therefore this technique is a useful aid in decongesting the Liver (see Fig. 5.19).

6. Knees Into Back Use palms initially to feel whether or not knee pressure is appropriate. One knee tonifies a Kyo area, while the other knee disperses Jitsu areas. Good hand support on shoulder and hip is essential. Strong Shiatsu can be given to the Bladder, Kidney and Small Intestine Channels using this technique. Please ensure that stationary pressure is applied perpendicular to the surface of the body (see Fig. 5.20).

This technique can be applied around the sacro-iliac and hip joints.

Fig. 5.19: Scapula loosening – sometimes called the 'chicken wing'

Fig. 5.20: Knees into back

7. Palms/Knees into Heart Channel extension

Fig. 5.21: Palms/knees into Heart Channel

SITTING POSITION

All these techniques could be done with the receiver sitting in a chair or sitting with legs outstretched, although more support will be required.

Apply two-handed pressure in a variety of positions across lower back and upper buttocks.

1. Child's Pose

Fig. 5.22: Child's pose

2. Palming the Back With firm support hand on shoulder, palm down each side of back. Support hand should be on the same side as the working hand, i.e. left shoulder supported, left side of back worked (see Fig. 5.23).

3. Neck Rotations The neck should be rotated in a posterior semi-circle and never through a full circle, which can damage the facet joints of the cervical vertebrae.

Neck rotations done well can relieve tension in the neck muscles and move Ki stagnation in the occiput, especially around BL-10 and GB-20 (see Fig. 5.24).

Fig. 5.23: Palming the back

Fig. 5.24: Neck rotations

Large Intestine Channel can be given maximum support in the arm and shoulder with this technique (see Fig. 5.25).

4. Forearm into Trapezius

Shoulder blades are folded back over fingertips. Inability to get under the shoulder blades can indicate GB Kyo or Jitsu: liver congestion on the right side, Stomach acidity on the left side (see Fig. 5.26).

5. Shoulder Blade Loosening

Fig. 5.25: Forearm into trapezius

Fig. 5.26: Scapula loosening

SHIATSU TO THE HARA AND CHEST

The Hara and Chest are very sensitive and protected parts of the body, and as such the receiver's confidence must be gained before Shiatsu can be administered there. However, under circumstances of mutual trust they can be extremely effective areas to work.

Generally the giver should be positioned on the right side of the receiver because many of the techniques, if done from this side, will facilitate the peristaltic movement of the bowel, particularly in the transverse colon where the bowel movement travels from right to left. Wave rocking is a good example of this.

1. Wave Rocking Kneeling, facing Hara. One hand on top of the other, knead the belly with a motion similar to a wave breaking upon the shore. This is good for moving Ki, and so should not be done on a very Kyo Hara (see Fig. 5.27).

2. Bowl Rotations Form an inverted bowl with both hands. Rotate the bowl's rim around client's belly, upon a central axis, in a clockwise direction (see Fig. 5.28).

3. Bowl Circling As above, for 2, but circle the axis of the bowl over the client's belly in a clockwise direction, thereby stretching the fascia more. This is excellent for sluggish bowels and poor abdominal circulation, but not suitable for very Kyo conditions (see Fig. 5.29).

Fig. 5.27: Wave rocking

The previous three techniques can also be done with one hand on the Hara, while the other gives support under the lumbar spine.

Gather the belly flesh to centre with both hands, from varying directions, but generally progressing in a clockwise direction (see Fig. 5.30).

4. Gathering to 'Centre'

Fig. 5.28: Bowl rotations

Fig. 5.29: Bowl circling

Fig. 5.30: Gathering to centre

All the previous techniques tend to disperse Jitsu. To tonify Kyo it is effective to simply hold perpendicular, stationary, focused touch, with palms or fingertips, provided there is a strong support hand nearby.

5. Sternal Cupping Place edges of both hands on either side of the sternum and lean in gently as receiver exhales (see Fig. 5.31).

Fig. 5.31: Sternal cupping

Chapter 6

Stretching

Stretching is a useful component of Shiatsu because it can:

- Improve flexibility
- Improve blood and lymphatic circulation
- Bring Channels closer to the surface
- Help disperse sections of a Channel and ease muscular tension
- Improve respiration by opening the rib cage

However, to apply stretch effectively, certain principles must be understood. A muscle consists of numerous contractile fibres bound together in parallel groups encased within a sheath of connective tissue. The sheath extends beyond the muscle fibres to form a strong fibrous cord known as a tendon, which attaches the muscle to the bone.

At rest, all muscles remain in a state of slight contraction called *tonus*. On receiving an impulse from a motor nerve, the muscle will contract further and shorten in length. On cessation of that impulse it will cease to shorten and return to a state of tonus.

Muscles usually work in pairs; for example the biceps muscle flexes the elbow and the triceps muscle extends the elbow. To allow the biceps to shorten and flex the elbow, the triceps must reduce its level of contraction, otherwise they would fight against each other and prevent movement from occurring. The muscle contracting to produce a movement is referred to as the *agonist* or *prime mover*, whereas the opposite muscle which relaxes to allow the movement is known as the *antagonist*. The degree of relaxation and lengthening in the antagonist is proportional to the strength and extent of contraction by the agonist. Therefore the more strongly the biceps contracts against resistance to flex the elbow joint, the more the triceps can relax and lengthen. Other muscles which increase in tonus to stabilize the rest of the body and prevent other joints from moving during agonist/antagonist interplay are known as *synergists* or *fixators*.

A muscle cannot be stretched as such because its fibres are not elastic, but actively contractile. Therefore the way to lengthen a muscle to achieve a greater range of movement is to reduce its tonus. This can be achieved by persuading the muscle's protective mechanisms to co-operate, which requires an understanding of the stretch reflex.

Fig. 6.1:
Muscle/tendon
structure

muscle belly

tendon
attaching muscle to bone

muscle

bundles of
muscle cells
(fasciculi)

muscle
cell

myofibril

myofilament
at rest

myofilament
contracted

THE STRETCH REFLEX

Nerves known as *muscle spindles* are connected in parallel to various muscle cells at intervals throughout the muscle. When the muscle lengthens, so do the muscle spindles. If the muscle is lengthened too quickly and too much, the muscle spindle will react by sending an impulse via the spinal cord telling the muscle to contract. This is a protective mechanism to prevent injury resulting from sudden overstretching, and is known as the stretch reflex.

When a person falls asleep in a sitting position, the head will relax forward, then jerk back up. This is an example of muscle spindle reflex within the muscles at the back of the neck (see Fig. 6.2).

Although the muscle spindle responds when the muscle is stretched unexpectedly, it does permit voluntary lengthening if it is slow and gradual.

Other nerve cells called tendon organs exist where the tendons join the muscle fibres. When the muscle is strongly contracted, the tendon organs are stretched, which initiates an impulse to the muscle telling it to relax. This is therefore the opposite of the stretch reflex insofar as muscle spindles cause muscles to contract when they are overstretched, whereas tendon organs relax muscles when they are overcontracted.

A muscle can be made to lengthen further than usual by first strongly contracting it to initiate a relaxation response from the tendon organs, and then lengthening the muscle slowly to avoid stimulating the muscle spindles (see Fig. 6.3).

This type of muscle lengthening is called *facilitated stretching* (or proprioceptive neuromuscular facilitation: PNF) and is the most effective way to increase flexibility. It is a major ingredient of the corrective exercise system known as Sotai.

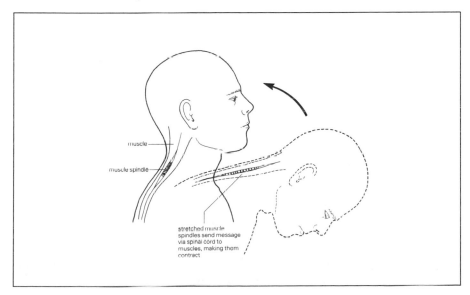

Fig. 6.2: Muscle spindles sending message to muscles at back of neck via spinal cord

Fig. 6.3(a): Prone lying: front thigh muscles contracted strongly against resistance showing tendon organs relaying messages to 'relax' via spinal cord

direction of resistance

direction of push

message to relax relayed from tendon organs to spinal cord

quadricep muscles contract

message from spinal cord sent to muscle fibres causing them to relax

tendon organ stretched

direction of pressure

quadricep muscles lengthened slowly

tendon organ relaxes

Fig. 6.3(b): Lengthen muscle slowly to avoid stimulating muscle spindles

There are three methods of lengthening muscles applicable within a Shiatsu session:

- Gravity stretching
- Passive assisted stretching
- Facilitated stretching

GRAVITY STRETCHING

Maximum support is given to anchor the body so that a specific muscle group can lengthen by surrendering to gravity (see Fig. 6.4).

With gravity stretching, the muscle spindle might initiate a muscle tonus for a few seconds, but the sustained opening of the muscle will pacify the spindles' impulses and allow more lengthening within two

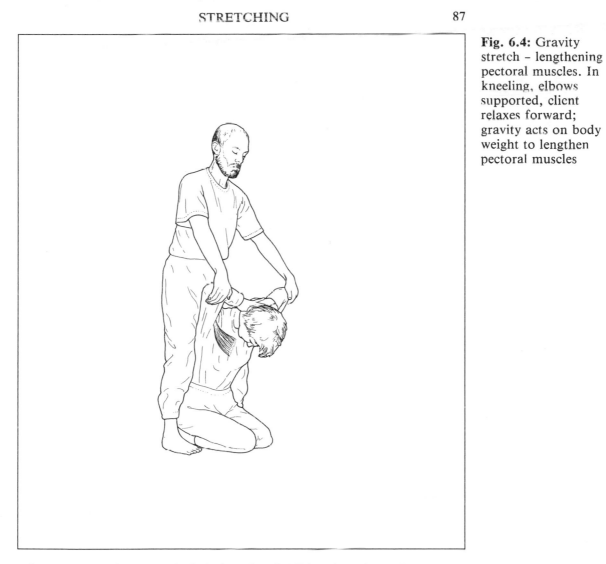

Fig. 6.4: Gravity stretch – lengthening pectoral muscles. In kneeling, elbows supported, client relaxes forward; gravity acts on body weight to lengthen pectoral muscles

minutes, assuming no pain is induced to inhibit relaxation. Slow, deep, rhythmical breathing helps.

PASSIVE ASSISTED STRETCHING

With passive assisted stretching the muscle being lengthened is very gently coaxed further with the help of a partner. This method operates by the same principle as gravity stretching, but is more effective (see Fig. 6.5).

FACILITATED STRETCHING

During facilitated stretching the muscle is lengthened to its comfortable limit and held for approximately 30 seconds. Then a static muscle

Fig. 6.5: Wrists on knees; improving respiration by opening rib cage with passive assisted stretching

direction of therapist's resistance and stretch

direction of push from recipient

Fig. 6.6: Facilitated stretch on hamstrings

contraction is held for 6–10 seconds. The muscle is then relaxed and a passive assisted stretch is applied, during which the muscle will lengthen further.

The example in Fig. 6.6 shows a facilitated stretch applied to the Hamstring muscle group.

Each type of stretch has its relevant applications:

- All improve flexibility, especially facilitated stretching;
- All improve blood and lymphatic circulation, especially facilitated stretching because the contraction followed by lengthening has a pumping and flushing effect on the blood and lymph vessels, which also helps the breakdown and elimination of waste products accumulated within the muscle;
- A gravity stretch, or mild passive assisted stretch will bring a

Channel section which is kyo (and thus deeper) to the surface;
- For dispersing Jitsu areas, a facilitated stretch is required because the contraction phase will tire and therefore soften the muscle, allowing the muscle, and any Channel flowing through it to open more easily during the passive assisted phase, thus aiding the dispersal of blocked or overconcentrated Ki;
- All types of stretch can be applied to improve respiration, by opening the ribs.

Caution: Facilitated stretching should not be done extensively on Kyo Channels or with very weak and debilitated receivers. One or two gentle facilitated stretches are permissable on Kyo sections of a Channel in order to 'wake up' the area, provided they are followed by sustained perpendicular pressure to tonify.

Figs. 6.7 and 6.8 will give you various examples of stretching techniques:

Improving Flexibility Using Facilitated Stretching

direction of resistance and stretch

direction of push from recipient

Fig. 6.7: Loosening hip adductors

**Improving Flexibility
Using Passive
Assisted Stretching**

Fig. 6.8: Side Neck stretch – this can be done as a facilitated stretch if extreme caution is observed

IMPROVING BLOOD AND LYMPHATIC CIRCULATION – USING 'CROSS FIBRE' PASSIVE ASSISTED STRETCHING

All the flexibility techniques previously mentioned improve the circulation of blood and lymph. However, an especially effective method for decongesting the by-products of muscle metabolism, and therefore reducing the soreness and stiffness commonly experienced

Fig. 6.9: Cross fibre stretch to a muscle belly

after strenuous exercise, is the 'cross fibre' passive assisted stretch. This technique is especially good for athletes and dancers.

A cross fibre stretch is a passive assisted stretch applied at right angles to the muscle fibres, a torsion which squeezes out stagnant waste products rather like wringing water out of a floor cloth (see Fig. 6.9).

Figs. 6.10 and 6.11 show a sequence of cross fibre stretching to relieve congestion in the thigh and calf.

(a)

(b)

Fig. 6.10: Quadriceps

Fig. 6.11: Calf muscles

(a)

(b)

Cross fibre stretching applied to the general musculature on either side of the vertebral column is excellent for loosening stiff backs. This can be done by stretching the muscle away from the spine in prone lying, or in sitting (see Fig. 6.12).

Cross fibre can be done very locally with thumbs or fingertips, 'pushing and pulling' the muscle fibres rythmically. This is known as *Kenbiki* technique (see Fig. 6.13).

Fig. 6.12: Sitting with forward twist

Fig. 6.13: Kenbiki applied to back muscles with fingertips. This technique can also be applied using the thumbs

BRINGING CHANNELS TO THE SURFACE

(Using gravity or passive assisted stretching)

Bringing a specific Channel to the surface within an arm or leg is simply achieved by placing the limb in a specific position. The required Channel can then be worked on more easily using less pressure. The stretch in itself 'opens' the Channel and encourages Ki to flow more smoothly. The following illustrations show these positions.

EXPOSING CHANNELS IN THE THIGH

Fig. 6.14: Channels in cross section viewed from above (left thigh)

POSTERIOR

Bladder

(Lung)

Kidney (Heart)

(Kidney)

MEDIAL

LATERAL

Liver

(Large Intestine)

ADDUCTOR LONGUS

Gall Bladder

FEMUR

FEMORAL ARTERY

(Heart Protector)

(Triple Heater)

(Small Intestine)

Stomach

Spleen

ANTERIOR

Channels in brackets = Masunaga's extensions to the Channels

Stretches in Supine

Fig. 6.15: Spleen

Fig. 6.16: Small Intestine extension

Fig. 6.17: Heart Protector extension

Fig. 6.18: Liver

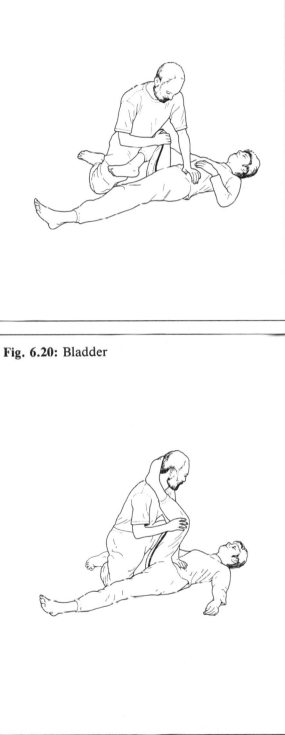

Fig. 6.19: Heart extension

Fig. 6.20: Bladder

Fig. 6.21: Lung extension

Fig. 6.22: Kidney extension

Fig. 6.23: Large Intestine extension

Fig. 6.24: Gall Bladder

Fig. 6.25: Triple Heater extension

Fig. 6.26: Stomach (A)

Fig. 6.27: Stomach (B) Variation for more flexible recipients

Stretches in Prone (below)

Fig. 6.28: Heart extension

Fig. 6.29: Bladder

Fig. 6.30: Lung extension

Fig. 6.31: Kidney extension

Fig. 6.32: Large Intestine extension

Fig. 6.33: Below left Gall bladder

Fig. 6.34: Below Triple Heater extension

Fig. 6.35: Stomach

Stretches in Side Lying

Fig. 6.36: Above Stomach

Fig. 6.37: Above right Spleen

Fig. 6.38: Right Bladder and Lung extension, and Kidney extension

Most of the lower leg Channels can be exposed with the same stretches as for the thigh. There is much less stretch occurring in the lower leg with these positions compared to the thigh, but the value lies in producing the optimum position to get at the Channels with correctly angled pressure.

EXPOSING CHANNELS IN THE ARM

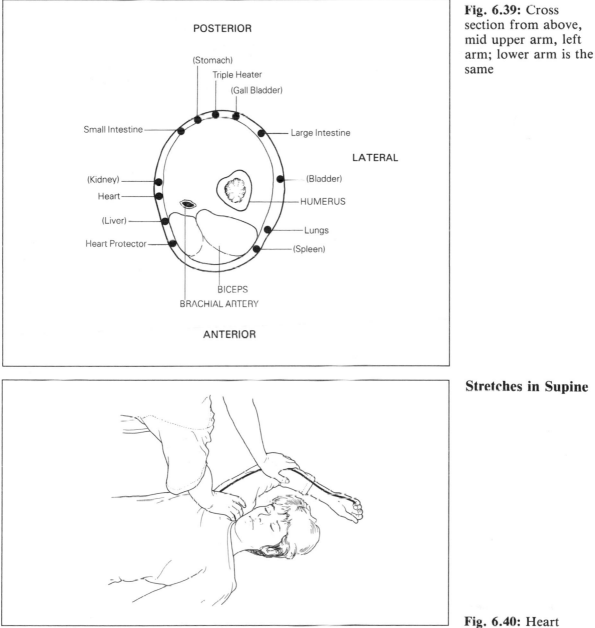

Fig. 6.39: Cross section from above, mid upper arm, left arm; lower arm is the same

Stretches in Supine

Fig. 6.40: Heart

Fig. 6.41: **Above** Liver extension

Fig. 6.42: **Above right** Heart Protector

Fig. 6.43: Spleen extension

Fig. 6.44: Lung (N.B. Recipient's hand should be palm up)

Fig. 6.45: Kidney/Bladder extensions (inner and outer edges of arms and forearms)

Fig. 6.46: Large Intestine

Fig. 6.47: Above Gall Bladder extension

Fig 6.48: Above right Triple Heater/Stomach extension

Fig. 6.49: Small Intestine

Fig. 6.50: Arm above head exposing Channels on posterior aspect of arm

LI
GB(ext)
TH
ST(ext)
SI

Stretches in Prone

Lu
SP(ext)
HP Liv(ext)
HT

Fig. 6.51: Arm by side exposing Channels on anterior aspect of arm

Stretches in Side Lying

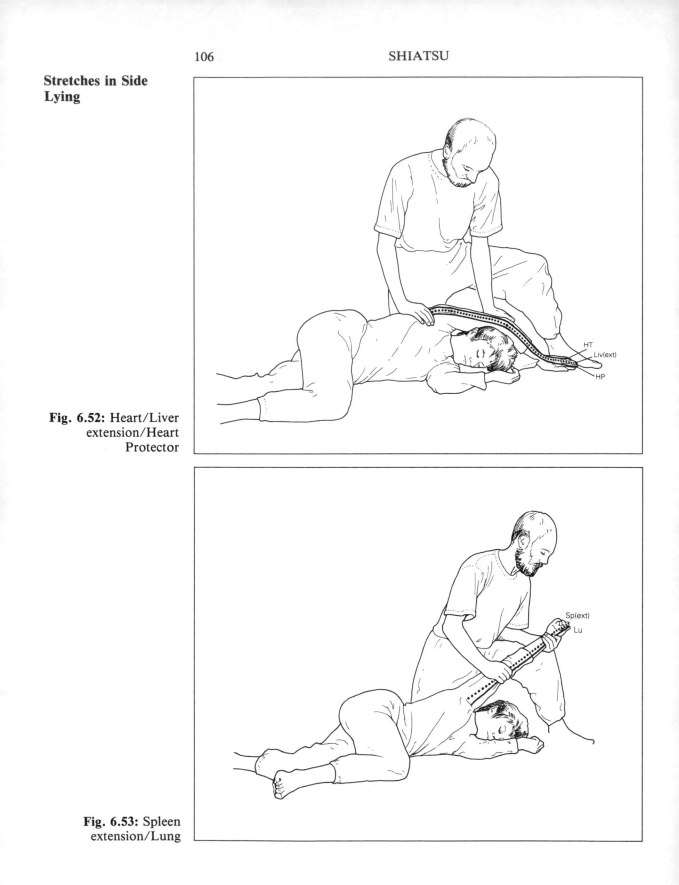

Fig. 6.52: Heart/Liver extension/Heart Protector

Fig. 6.53: Spleen extension/Lung

Fig. 6.54: Kidney/Bladder extensions

Fig. 6.55: Large intestine

Fig. 6.56: Gall Bladder extension/Triple Heater/Stomach extension

Fig. 6.57: Small Intestine

With a little imagination, you can adapt the supine stretches for use in sitting (for example Fig 6.58). **Stretches in Sitting**

Fig. 6.58: Heart

EXPOSING CHANNELS IN TORSO

Generally, we simply have the receiver lying on his or her back to expose the Channels on the front of the torso, and have them lie on their front or side to expose the Channels on the back of the torso (see Fig. 6.59).

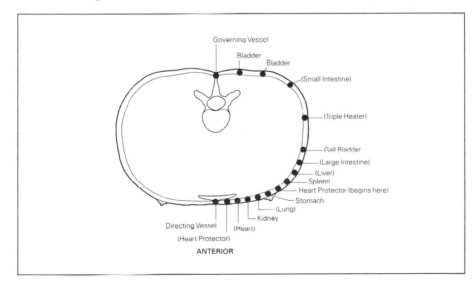

Fig. 6.59: Cross section through torso at nipple level, viewed from above

EXPOSING CHANNELS IN NECK

Fig. 6.60: Cross section through mid neck from above

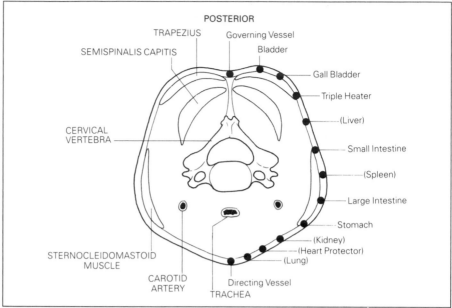

Fig. 6.61: Anterior aspect of neck

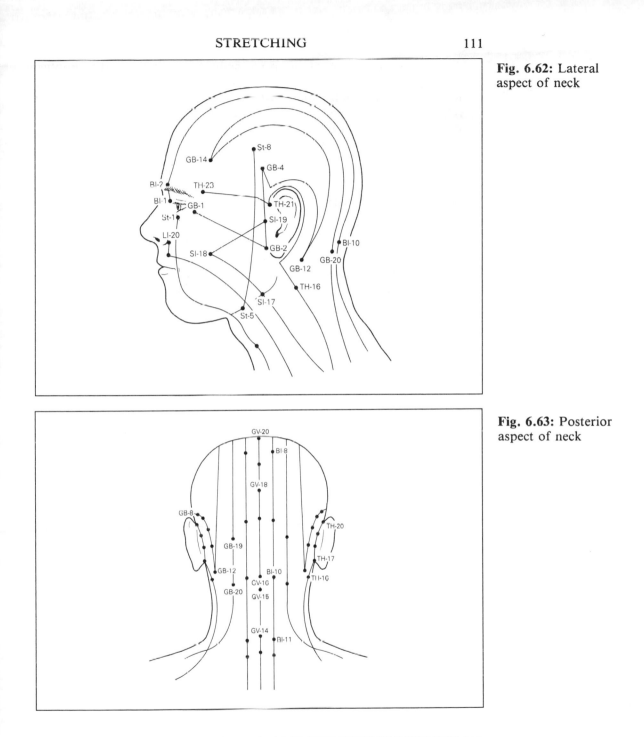

Fig. 6.62: Lateral aspect of neck

Fig. 6.63: Posterior aspect of neck

DISPERSING JITSU CHANNELS AND RELIEVING MUSCULAR TENSION USING FACILITATED STRETCHING

All the techniques described to improve flexibility and aid blood and lymphatic circulation can be used to disperse a Jitsu Channel section and relieve tense muscles. Similarly a facilitated stretch could be applied to many of the Channel opening positions. Bear in mind that tense muscles have an underlying cause which must be dealt with for maximum positive change. For example, tense shoulder and neck muscles may be due to emotional factors, or postural factors such as hip misalignment or a weak lumbar region.

OPENING THE RIB CAGE USING PASSIVE ASSISTED STRETCHING

Many people lack vitality simply because they fail to breathe to their full potential. This is partly the result of poor posture arising from a sedentary lifestyle, and partly due to being out of touch with their Hara – which is exacerbated by a sedentary lifestyle. Being out of touch with Hara immediately raises the centre of gravity so that the breathing becomes focused in the upper chest. It also makes one less able to maintain a state of relaxation in the face of routine stress factors, and more prone to emotional ups and downs. All these factors cause the breathing to be more shallow, quicker and more erratic.

It helps therefore, to assist the receiver to relax and become aware of their centre. Good general Shiatsu does this effectively. However, direct work on opening the rib cage can allow the receiver to experience what a deep breath is, maybe for the first time (see Figs 6.64 and 6.65).

Fig. 6.64: Supine lying: lower rib press to extend exhalation, so that receiver automatically stretches ribs on resultant increased inhalation, thus encouraging awareness of breath in lower rib cage. Can be progressed by positioning arms over head

In the previous two examples a resistance could be applied during the inhalation phase. On release of pressure, the ribs will expand greatly and suddenly, bringing maximum air into the lungs.

Caution: This should be avoided in cases of high blood pressure, suspected weak ribs or asthma.

Fig. 6.65: Above left Supine lying: diagonal rib press; this and the previous technique can be done lying face down applying pressure to the back of the rib cage

Fig. 6.66: Above In sitting; 'Drape', using palms in back

Fig. 6.67: Left In sitting; 'Drape', using knees in back (more powerful, can be painful)

Fig. 6.68: In sitting; receiver lies forward with arms supported by giver's thighs. Pressure applied to back with forearms

Fig. 6.69: In sitting; giver stands and stretches receiver's arms overhead, simultaneously easing thigh into back

Fig. 6.70: In side lying; 'Bow' stretch (also an extreme stretch for the Stomach Channel)

A WORD ABOUT LIGAMENTS

A common misconception is that it is desirable to loosen the ligaments surrounding a joint to improve the range of movement a joint can

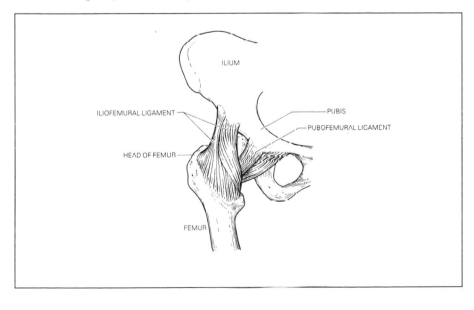

Fig. 6.71: Ligaments around the hip joint

perform. Nothing could be further from the truth. The range of movement any given joint is capable of is limited by tight muscles. The ligaments exist to support and stabilize the joint, thereby preventing excessive movement, or movement in undesirable directions. They literally strap the joint in place.

The ligaments have no elasticity and no ability to contract, being made of bands of connective tissue. If you stretch a ligament you will merely weaken it and make it more susceptible to tearing. Once stretched or torn, ligaments are extremely slow to repair because they have a very poor blood supply. Loose ligaments around a joint can render the joint liable to recurrent dislocation, as is common with the shoulder joint. Furthermore, the opposing joint surfaces can become mismatched, resulting in uneven wear and tear, and the consequent early onset of osteoarthritis.

A strong but flexible, elongatable musculature, with strong, firm ligaments is the ideal. Weak, loose muscles and loose ligaments are detrimental. However, there are circumstances when the joints are too tightly bound and congested, and require gentle mobilization.

PART 2

SHIATSU THERAPY AND ORIENTAL MEDICINE

Shiatsu is essentially a tactile, practical method for promoting health. One can practise Shiatsu with relatively little understanding of its theoretical basis. However, a solid grasp of its roots in Oriental Medicine will supplement intuitive skills and give an added depth of insight and confidence.

The application of the Kyo/Jitsu method in diagnosis and treatment can be very effective. However, this method in itself does not indicate the cause of an imbalance, nor the factors underlying the symptoms. Oriental Medicine provides a theoretical framework for understanding how physical and mental disharmonies originate and manifest.

The purpose of this section, therefore, is to present the fundamentals of Traditional Oriental Medicine. It includes those areas of Oriental Medicine important for a thorough knowledge of the causative patterns of disease and their alleviation through Shiatsu. Only such thorough knowledge will avoid the kind of misunderstanding and over-generalization to which Oriental Medicine is sometimes subject.

In practice, a Shiatsu therapist will tend to rely either more upon sensitivity and intuition, or upon reason and knowledge. The former type of practitioner will depend less upon their theoretical understanding and more upon their sensitivity to the flow of Ki. The latter type of practitioner will use a wider range of diagnostic skills and more frequently employ classical Tsubos. However, to rely exclusively on one approach or the other will limit the effectiveness of the treatment given. A well-rounded practitioner is one who realizes the full potential of Shiatsu through developing both sensitivity and theoretical insight. They are the practitioners who will ensure that Shiatsu therapy maintains a prominent position in natural medicine.

Chapter 7

Tao and Yin/Yang

TAO

Chinese Medicine evolved alongside the ancient philosophy of the *Tao*. The Tao literally means a 'way' or a 'path'. To Taoists it came to mean 'The Way of the Universe'. One of its many observations is that all phenomena are embraced by the Tao and so function ultimately as a whole. All things in life can only be understood in relation to life in its entirety.

Because the omnipresence of the Tao is a difficult concept to grasp, it is seen as 'elusive and intangible',[1] 'dim and dark' to mind and language. As the great sage Lao Tzu tells us in the Taoist classic, the *Tao Te Ching*:

The Tao that can be told is not the eternal Tao.
The name that can be named is not the eternal name.[2]

The Tao is that 'irreducible dimension of the Real'[3] which cannot be known or described through the analytical tool of words: it must be apprehended through direct experience – it must be lived. It is at once both hidden to one's mind and yet intimate with one's Being.

The Tao serves, sustains and yields to, rather than governs and directs:

The ten thousand things depend on it: it holds nothing back.
It fulfils its purpose silently and makes no claim.[4]

Embracing all things and rejecting nothing, the Tao is a way of expressing an Ultimate Reality which 'does not show greatness, and therefore is truly great'. Instead of *exerting* power like the God of the early Judaeo-Christian religions, it *contains* power like 'an empty vessel. It is used, but never filled.'[5] Without effort, the Tao assumes the role of a unifying principle only by virtue of its omnipresence:

Heaven's net casts wide.
Though its meshes are coarse, nothing slips through.[6]

Lao Tzu admonishes us to be 'at one with the Tao'. In Shiatsu, the practitioner should allow him or herself to *yield* his or her energy to the recipient in an effortless way; without straining or tensing, and without using overt physical force. Instead, gravity and body weight are used to apply pressure to the recipient, and the practitioner becomes, like the Tao, an 'empty vessel'.

From the perspective of the Tao, the practitioner will see the patient's disharmony as a part of the bodymind which has become detached from its true totality. The practitioner re-establishes harmony simply by helping the patient regain their innate oneness. 'The Tao of Heaven does not strive, and yet it overcomes.'

Disease in the Taoist vision is therefore seen as a situation where the individual is at some level 'out of step' with the dynamic, ever-changing, yet harmonious balance of Nature. This may be contrasted with Western scientific medicine which views disease as an invasive force unrelated and alien to the whole. In contrast, the Taoist believes that 'those who would conquer must yield'.[7]

The Tao is the source of all order; a cosmic order which is not static but organic in nature. It is complete in itself, and requires no doctrine in order to exist.

> You cannot improve it.
> If you try to change it, you will ruin it.
> If you try to hold it, you will lose it.[8]

The Tao guides without Laws or Commandments, and maintains harmony through 'Virtue', by which 'all things are nourished'. 'Virtue' is living according to the Tao:

> Creating without claiming,
> Doing without taking credit,
> Guiding without interfering.[9]

YIN/YANG

Yin/Yang are inseparable from the Tao: they are the two hands through which the Tao manifests and orders creation. Although they represent two polar antagonistic tendencies, they are complementary and interdependent. Everything in creation contains within it a Yin and Yang aspect; it is only in a relative sense that one thing is more Yin or Yang than another. The Yin/Yang dyad can be used to understand the relationship between any two structures, functions or processes. It forms the basis of Oriental Medicine.

The Yin aspect of a phenomenon is the structural and substantial; its Yang aspect is the active and energetic. Yin is therefore equated with the condensed and consolidated, dominated by the gravity of Earth. Yang mobilizes and expands, centrifugal in movement, associated with non-material existence or 'Heaven'.

Yin is like the ovum; Yang like the sperm. Yin remains a potential energy until it is activated by Yang. Thus, 'Heaven' acts on Earth, and Earth nourishes 'Heaven'. The two are interdependent; they flow into and contain each other, as illustrated in their symbol:

In terms of gender, Yin is considered to be more feminine, and Yang more masculine. However, just as it is incorrect to say a particular food is either Yin or Yang, it is equally misinformed to say that a woman is Yin and a man is Yang. All things are an interplay of both forces.

In the case of the human sexes, it is interesting to note that although women are outwardly more Yin, they contain within a more masculine unconscious which Carl Jung called the Animus. In turn, men possess a more feminine unconscious called the Anima. This is an example of the profound interdependence inherent in Yin/Yang.

Fig. 7.1: Yin/Yang

YIN/YANG IN THE HUMAN BODY

In terms of bodily energetics, Chinese Medicine has selected four important Yin/Yang polarities and termed them the 'Eight Principles'. The Eight Principles provide the basic categories for the classification of bodily disharmonies.

Interior/Exterior

The first two Principles provide a concept of bodily location in terms of Yin/Yang: these are Interior/Exterior. The Interior of the body is its more dense, Yin region, where the internal organs are located. The Exterior includes the relatively more superficial, Yang layers of the body; namely the skin and muscles. It is the more Yang role of the Exterior to protect the Interior. The Exterior protects the body from pathogenic factors such as Cold and Dampness which tend to invade the body from the outside. Diseases which are due to pathogenic invasion are called 'Exterior conditions'. These types of conditions always require Shiatsu treatment which is dispersing in style, in order to help the body drive out the unwanted pathogens.

Problems which arise from within, whether chronic or acute, are in turn called 'Interior conditions'. They may require either tonification or dispersal, depending on the particular condition involved.

Although not included among the 'Eight Principles', another polarity of body location is superior/inferior. Because Yang describes upward-moving energy and Yin downward, the upper parts of the body are more Yang and the lower more Yin. The brain, at the more Yang superior pole of the body, is concerned with more rarefied, subtle and Yang phenomena; namely nervous stimuli and thought. The intestines, in a relatively more Yin inferior position, accordingly deal with more coarse, dense and Yin phenomena.

Hot/Cold   The second Eight Principle polarity is Hot/Cold. Normal body function requires internal warmth not only for comfort, but for its many different transformative functions. Processes of warming and transformation (e.g. of food into Blood) belong to the Yang function of the body. They find their source in the 'Gate of Vitality' ('Ming Men') provided by the Yang (energetic) aspect of the Kidneys and located near the Tsubo Governor Vessel-4.

In contrast, it is the role of the Yin of the body to cool, calm and moisten. The body's Yin is derived from the Yin aspect of the Kidneys and from the Stomach, which, because of its role in digestion, is the source of the Body Fluids.

When, for a variety of possible reasons, the body's warming functions are over-stimulated, often at the expense of its cooling ones, a Hot condition arises. The signs of internal Heat include thirst, possible fever, restlessness, a rapid pulse, a red face and tongue, and scanty, dark urine. They indicate a relative excess of Yang in the body. If on the other hand, the body's warming functions become impaired, a Cold condition arises, involving signs which include chilliness, a lack of thirst, a pale face and tongue, and abundant, clear urine. They indicate a relative excess of Yin.

Full/Empty   The Eight Principle categories of Full/Empty provide another important way of assessing bodily condition, and are particularly relevant to the practice of Shiatsu. A Full condition is one which is characterized by a certain type of excess. It is more Yang in nature. An Empty condition is characterized by deficiency, and is more Yin in nature. The signs of a Full condition include a sudden, acute onset of symptoms with pain made worse by pressure, profuse sweating, irritability, and a strong voice. The signs of an Empty condition include chronic disease with pain alleviated by pressure, slight sweating, listlessness, and a weak voice. In reality, most disharmonies include signs of both a Full and Empty character, although one of the two usually predominate.

In Shiatsu, Full/Empty conditions may be perceived directly through palpation of the body surface in both diagnosis and treatment, and are classified according to the terms Kyo/Jitsu.

Jitsu signifies a Full condition and is characterized by hardness, stiffness, pain aggravated by pressure, and possibly swelling, redness and heat. It indicates the presence either of stagnant Ki (causing stiffness), stagnant Blood (often causing swelling), excess Yang (generating heat) or excess Cold (producing pain and cramping). Although it is difficult to generalize, Jitsu conditions are most commonly found along the Liver, Gall Bladder and Stomach Channels. Any Channels or Tsubos exhibiting a Jitsu condition always require treatment which is dispersing in style.

Kyo signifies an Empty condition and is characterized by flaccidity, weakness, mild pain which is alleviated by pressure, and pale, cold skin. Stiffness or hardness of muscles which seem to lack Ki can also be Kyo.

Emptiness of Ki and/or Blood commonly leads to areas of the body such as the Hara exhibiting a loss of muscular tone, and showing a lack of resistance to pressure. Emptiness of Yang in the body will add paleness and coldness to these signs. Although, again, it is difficult to generalize, Kyo conditions are most commonly felt along the Kidney and Spleen Channels. A Kyo condition always requires treatment which is tonifying in style.

Yin/Yang Balance

The last two Eight Principle categories are Yin and Yang themselves, and generally serve to summarize the ones we have already discussed.

There are three Yin/Yang diagnostic classifications which are found in practice: these are (1) Empty Yang; (2) Excess Yang; and (3) Empty Yin. Excess Yin is not generally considered to be a common occurrence, as it results only from exposure to extremes of cold.

When Yang becomes excessive, the body generates heat and becomes hyperactive. This is Excess Yang. Alternatively, a Hot condition may also arise because of a lack of cool, moist Yin energy in the body, allowing the Yang to predominate and so generate heat and dryness. This is Empty Yin. The following graphs illustrate and compare Empty Yang with Excess Yang, as well as the important distinction between Excess Yang and Empty Yin.

Fig. 7.2: A graph of Yin/Yang combinations

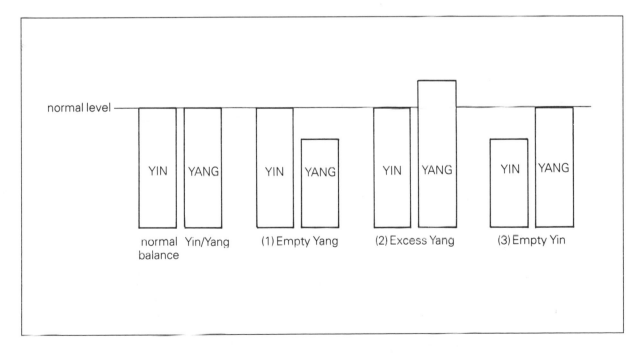

Let us now summarize these three basic states of bodily disharmony by comparing their signs and symptoms.

Empty Yang	*Excess Yang*	*Empty Yin*
tired	restless	restless but underlying weakness
sleeps heavily	can't get to sleep/restless sleep	gets to sleep but wakes frequently
cold	hot	hot hands and feet
cold day and night	hot day and night	hot mainly during afternoon/night
no thirst	strong thirst	thirst mainly during afternoon/night
pale face	red face	red cheeks ('malar flush')
pale tongue with white coating	red tongue with yellow coating	bright red thin tongue (no coating)
copious, clear urine	scanty, dark urine	scanty, dark urine
loose stools	constipated with possible pain	dry stools with no pain
listless	agitated	anxious
unconfident	arrogant	defensive
apathetic	driven	over-extended

Finally, Yin/Yang is used to classify the internal organs into pairs, each pair sharing the same Element. The Yin (or 'Zang') organs are those which are relatively more solid in structure. They 'store the precious Substances' (i.e. the Essence, Ki, Blood and pure Body Fluids). The Yang (or 'Fu' organs) are considered 'hollow workshop organs', and are responsible for the transportation and excretion of bodily substances. Each pair of organs are interdependent. Although the most important body functions belong to the Yin organs, the Channels of both the Yin and Yang organs are of equal importance in Shiatsu therapy.

Element	Yin (Zang) Organ	Yang (Fu) Organ
Water	Kidneys	Bladder
Wood	Liver	Gall Bladder
Fire	Heart	Small Intestines
	Heart Governor	Triple heater
Earth	Spleen	Stomach
Metal	Lungs	Large Intestines

NOTES

1. *Tao Te Ching* by Lao Tzu, translated by Gia-Fu Feng and Jane English, Vintage Books, 1972, ch. 21.
2. *Tao Te Ching*, ch. 1.
3. *Survey of Traditional Chinese Medicine*, by Claude Larre, Jean Schatz and Elisabeth Rochat de la Vallee, translated by Sarah Elizabeth Stang, Institut Ricci, Paris, and Traditional Acupuncture Institute, U.S.A., 1986, p.39.
4. *Tao Te Ching*, ch. 24.
5. *Tao Te Ching*, ch. 4.
6. *Tao Te Ching*, ch. 73.
7. *Tao Te Ching*, ch. 61.
8. *Tao Te Ching*, ch. 29.
9. *Tao Te Ching*, ch. 51.

Chapter 8

The Vital Substances

At the basis of Oriental Medicine are the four fundamental Substances of the bodymind: Ki, Blood, 'Essence' (Jing) and Body Fluids. The word 'substance' is possibly misleading, as they should really be viewed as vital forces, each varying in the amount of actual 'substance' it possesses. Of the four, Ki is the most rarefied and active; hardly a 'substance' at all. Blood is relatively more material in form, yet helps the Heart to house the Mind. The Essence is the most concentrated of the vital substances – a type of 'essential energy'.[1] The Body Fluids are also material in form, yet even they possess energetic importance.

'Mind' (Shen) may be considered a type of Ki – the most refined of all. 'Shen' has often been translated as 'Spirit', but the Shen does not in fact refer to the primarily 'spiritual' aspect of an individual. Shen is something much more fundamental: it is one's day-to-day consciousness and all that this entails. It embraces thoughts, feelings, dreams and perceptions of every possible kind; not just those of a 'spiritual' nature. The Mind will be discussed in detail in Chapter 13.

The concept of Ki   Ki (Qi in Chinese) is generally translated as 'energy'. However, a look at the Chinese character for Ki reveals that it has two different aspects: a component which represents a 'vapour' or 'gas' and one that means 'rice'. These symbols express its material and immaterial manifestations. Also, the vapour represents the air we breathe and the rice, the food we eat; together they form bodily Ki.

Ki forms the very basis of all phenomena in the universe and affords a continuum between crude substance and subtle, invisible force. It animates and moves, changing constantly, gathering and dispersing in life's perpetual play.

The concept of bodily Ki is relatively more specific but no less fundamental. According to the *Nan Jing* (AD 100), 'Ki is the root of a human being.' It governs all the body's processes, both physical and mental, and thus appears as different types of Ki varying in location and function.

ESSENCE

'Essence' or 'Jing' is Ki at its most dense. It is formed at conception and nourishes the foetus during pregnancy, depending on the mother's Kidneys for sustenance. One might think of it as genetic in origin. This so-called 'Pre-Heaven Essence' accounts for individual constitutional strength and resistance to disease. Because it is inherited from one's parents, it is generally fixed in quantity and quality. However, overwork, poor diet and excessive sexual activity over a long period will contribute to the early depletion of Pre-Heaven Essence. On the other hand, it can be strengthened through special ways of cultivating Ki such as Tai Ji Quan, Qi Gong and Yoga.

The term 'Post-Heaven Essence' is given to the Essence which is extracted from food and refined by the Stomach and Spleen after birth. It replenishes the Pre-Heaven Essence stored in the Kidneys, and together they produce the generalized Essence which, due to its fluid nature, is able to circulate throughout the body.

The Essence has a number of functions all concerned with growth, reproduction and development, as well as sexual maturation, conception and pregnancy. It is said to fill 'The Sea of Bone Marrow', consisting not only of the bones but of the brain, spinal cord and teeth as well.

The Essence therefore determines proper growth and development of the entire individual, particularly of the bones, teeth and hair. It also provides the basis for normal brain development. According to the *Nei Ching*, the Essence of a man follows an eight-year cycle, while the Essence of a woman follows a seven-year cycle. In this way, the Essence controls the development of sexual characteristics, reproductive function and fertility. Without the Essence, conception and pregnancy would be impossible. Finally, it determines the natural decline of sexual energy and fertility in the ageing process.

As the Essence is stored in the Kidneys, it interacts closely with the Yin, Yang and Ki of the Kidneys.

Picture the Kidneys as a cauldron full of water: The fire under the cauldron is produced by the Kidney-Yang and the 'Gate of Vitality' ('Ming Men') located at the Tsubo Governor Vessel-4; the water contained by the cauldron may be thought of as the Kidney-Essence and Kidney-Yin; and the steam produced by the heating of the water represents the Kidney-Ki which results from the process. Kidney-Ki thus ascends to the Lungs, which are responsible for its dispersal around the body (see Fig. 8.1).

In short, the Essence provides the Kidney-Yin with the necessary substance to form Kidney-Ki through the warming action of Kidney-Yang.

Finally, due to its 'genetic' nature, the Essence accounts for our underlying constitutional strength and resistance to disease. If the Essence is deficient at birth, or becomes depleted later in life, a number of possible problems may manifest. Those problems related to growth,

Fig. 8.1: Kidney 'cauldron'

reproduction and development include retarded growth in children, malformation of bones, infertility, repeated miscarriage, loose teeth, loss of hair and premature ageing. Those problems directly involving the Kidneys include lower back pain, poor sexual vitality and hearing problems. If a deficiency of Essence affects the 'Sea of Bone Marrow' (which includes the brain), there may be a lack of concentration and memory as well as dizziness and tinnitus (ringing in the ears). In a general sense, the Essence contributes to the vitality of Ki and clarity of the mind; a deficiency will mean susceptibility to disease and mental fatigue.

The strength of the Essence may be assessed from the patient's medical history. A further sign of poor constitution is the absence of complete and detached earlobes: if the lobes are attached to the skin or virtually absent, it may be taken as another indication that the Essence should be cultivated.

KI

There are a number of types of Ki, all with different bodily and energetic functions. Its functions include the transformation of food into energy and Blood, the transportation of Fluids, holding the Organs in place, and the protecting and warming of the body.

The following explanation of the various types of Ki illustrates the detail with which Oriental Medicine explains the transformation of Ki within the body.

The first type of Ki is Original Ki. Original Ki stems directly from the Essence; in fact, it is Essence in the form of Ki, and can be considered our constitutional energy. Original Ki is the motivating force behind every function in the body. It acts as a catalyst for the creation of all the other types of Ki, as well as for the transformation of Food into Blood. It thus forms the basis of bodily vitality and endurance.

Original Ki is the foundation of the Hara and resides at its very centre, in the Gate of Vitality. The Gate of Vitality lies below the navel, between the Kidneys, and is the source-point of the body's energy and warmth. It is associated with two main Tsubos: Directing Vessel-6 (the lower 'Sea of Ki') and Governing Vessel-4 ('Ming Men' or 'Gate of Vitality'). Tonification of these points will directly reinforce the Gate of Vitality and the Original Ki. Like the Essence, the Original Ki is closely connected to the Kidneys, and provides the basis of Kidney-Ki. However, it is the job of the Triple Heater to spread the Original Ki from the Gate of Vitality to the internal Organs and their twelve main channels, where it surfaces at the Source Points.

Food Ki is produced by the Stomach and Spleen through the transformation of food into energy. However, Food Ki cannot be utilized by the body until it rises to the chest and combines with air to form Gathering Ki. It is the Spleen's function to raise the Food Ki to the chest where, with the help of the Original Ki, Food Ki is transformed into Blood.

Gathering Ki, also called Chest Ki, is a combination of Food Ki and Air Ki. It is a more refined and rarefied form of Ki than Food Ki and is therefore more easily utilized by the body. It vitalizes the Lungs and Heart, gives strength to the voice and invigorates the circulation of blood. It is located at the Tsubo Directing Vessel-17 (the upper 'Sea of Ki') and may be tonified through stimulation of this point.

Gathering Ki gives rise to True Ki under the motivating power of Original Ki. True Ki is the last stage in the transformation of Ki from its relatively crude state as Original Ki. Like Gathering Ki, True Ki is governed by the Lungs, the main function of which is to control Ki as a whole. True Ki manifests in two different forms; Nutritive Ki and Defensive Ki.

Nutritive Ki circulates in the Channels and blood vessels and, together

Fig. 8.2: Transformation of Ki

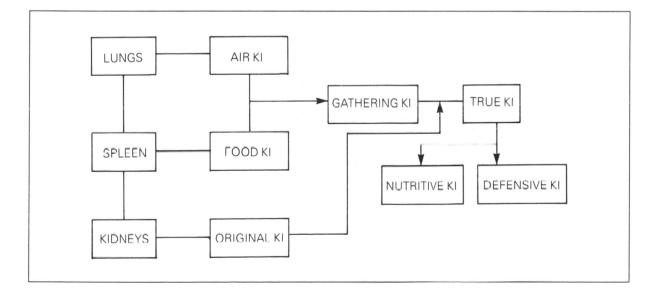

with the blood, supplies the body with nourishment. Defensive Ki is more Yang in relation to Nutritive Ki and circulates around the periphery of the body in the space between the muscles and skin. It acts as a protective barrier to the external world. Whereas Nutritive Ki is located in the interior and nourishes the body, Defensive Ki flows on the Exterior and protects it.

Whenever the body is exposed to external pathogenic factors such as Heat, Cold, Wind and Damp, the Defensive Ki acts like a shield to block their invasive power. It has the further function of warming and moistening the skin and muscles, opening and closing the pores, and therefore of regulating body temperature.

Both the skin and the muscles are controlled by the Lungs. It is therefore not surprising that a weakness of Lung Ki can lead to a weakness of Defensive Ki, and make one more susceptible to colds and flu. However, it should be noted that the Defensive Ki is also supported by the Kidney-Ki and is nourished by the Spleen and Stomach.

BLOOD

The Blood has wider connotations in Oriental Medicine than in Western understanding. Apart from transporting the body's nourishment, the Blood also plays a role in housing the Mind.

The process of Blood formation begins with the Spleen, which transforms and refines food and liquid into Food Ki, the basis of Blood. From the Spleen Food Ki is raised by the Lungs to the Heart. Here, with the help of the Original Ki, it is transformed into Blood. Although the Spleen is the origin of Blood, it is the Heart which 'governs' the Blood, mainly because it is responsible for its circulation. However, the Spleen also plays an important role in keeping the Blood in the blood vessels; it 'controls' the Blood.

Apart from providing the Original Ki necessary for Blood formation, the Kidneys play a further role through their production of the Bone Marrow, which also contributes to the manufacture of Blood.

The Liver is not directly involved in the production of Blood but is responsible for the storage of Blood during times of sleep and rest. When the body is in a horizontal position, a large proportion of the Blood goes to the Liver to be stored, and only circulates again when the body is active.

Finally, it should be noted that the Blood has a close interdependent relationship with the Ki. Not only is Ki crucial to Blood formation, but is also necessary for the circulation of Blood through the vessels: the Ki moves the Blood.

BODY FLUIDS

Body Fluids are the product of food and drink which have been transformed and separated by the Spleen and Stomach. The 'clean' fluids are transported to the Lungs. The Lungs then disperse them around the body and under the skin, as well as down to the Kidneys.

The 'dirty' portion of the fluids we take are further refined by the Small Intestines; the pure portion goes to the Bladder for its excretion as perspiration and urine, and the impure portion is excreted by the Large Intestines. Some water is reabsorbed by the Large Intestines and goes to the Bladder, mainly for excretion.

The Spleen is the most important organ in relation to the Body Fluids, as it ensures that the pure fluids move upwards for dissemination by the Lungs, and the impure fluids move downwards for excretion by the Bladder. When a Ki- or Yang-deficient Spleen fails to transform fluids as it should, an excessive build-up of Body Fluids will lead to Damp or Phlegm accumulation. It is usually necessary to treat the Spleen in this instance.

The Kidneys also play a vital role in the control of Body Fluids. First, they help to remove impure fluids from the body. Secondly, they vaporize some of the fluids they receive and send them up to the Lungs, helping to keep the Lungs moist. Finally, they supply the Bladder, their paired Organ, with the necessary Ki to transform fluids into sweat and urine.

The Lungs 'dominate the Water passages' through their function of dispersing and descending – dispersing Body Fluids throughout the body to the space beneath the skin, and descending them to the Kidneys. (Note that the Kidneys and Lungs have a reciprocal relationship: the Kidneys vaporize the Body Fluids and send them up to the Lungs for dispersal; the Lungs send down Body Fluids to the Kidneys for their excretion.)

Finally, the Organ of Triple Heater plays an important supportive role in the physiology of Body Fluids. It is said in *The Yellow Emperor's Classic* that 'The Triple Heater is the official in charge of irrigation, and controls the water passages.' The Upper Heater, likened to a 'mist', helps the Lungs in its dispersing and descending functions, as well as the Spleen in its job of 'raising the Food-Ki'. The Middle Heater, compared to a 'muddy pool', assists the Stomach in churning the fluids and sending the 'dirty' portion downwards. The Lower Heater is like a 'drainage ditch' because it helps the Kidneys, Bladder and Small Intestines separate and excrete fluids. It is the Triple Heater which orchestrates these many processes, and ensures the availability of the Original Ki necessary to effect them.

Thus, the Body Fluids are like the Blood: both are closely dependent upon the Ki for their transformation and transportation. In turn, they support the Ki through nourishing and moistening the Organs which produce, disseminate and regulate Ki.

Chapter 9

The Causes of Disease

The causes of disease in Oriental Medicine are categorized according to those which are Internal (i.e. emotional); those which are External (i.e. climatic); and those which are miscellaneous.

THE INTERNAL CAUSES OF DISEASE

In Oriental Medicine there is a direct relationship between the emotional life of a person and their physical health. Each internal Organ is closely associated with a range of associated emotions. The Organs dominate the expression of particular emotions and their function is in turn affected by them. For example, a disharmony of the Lungs will lead to sadness and melancholy; conversely, always feeling sad will weaken the Lungs. Thus, in diagnosis, little distinction is ultimately made between the mind and the body. Remembering this, it is easy to understand how certain emotions can play a role in the causation of disease.

The seven basic emotions which make up the Internal Causes of Disease are:

- Fear
- Anger
- Joy
- Shock or Fright
- Worry
- Pensiveness
- Sadness

These terms are broad categories and include a wide range of associated feelings. In normal circumstances they play a generally positive role in the life of bodymind. They only exert a negative influence when they become too intense or dominate the psyche over a long period of time.

Fear An appropriate sense of instinctive fear is important for survival. However, excessive or prolonged fear makes the Ki descend and drains the Kidneys. In particular, fear depletes the Kidneys of Yin, causing Heat in the Heart and related emotions such as anxiety and insecurity.

Anger is sometimes necessary to exert one's authority. However, **Anger** excessive and inappropriate anger make the Ki rise and causes Stagnation or Heat in the Liver. Headaches, indigestion and other problems commonly result. The term Anger here may include a number of associated feelings such as frustration, irritability and resentment.

Joy in general is naturally beneficial to one's emotional well-being. **Joy** What can be damaging is over-excitement and an abnormal degree of mental stimulation, both of which are forms of excessive 'Joy'. This type of excessive Joy slows down the Ki.

Mental shock scatters the Ki and adversely affects both the Kidneys and **Shock** Heart. The Ki of the Heart is rapidly weakened and requires the Kidney-Essence to support it. This in turn puts a strain on the Kidneys.

Worry and pensiveness (excessive thinking) are said to 'knot' the Ki, **Worry and** thereby disrupting the flow of Ki in the spleen and, to some extent, the **Pensiveness** Lungs. Because the Spleen houses Thought, it is particularly affected by thinking which is obsessive and fraught with over-concern. The Spleen's central role in digestion becomes disrupted and Dampness accumulates in the body. The Lungs react to worry by causing difficulty in breathing.

The Lungs when in a state of harmony are the source of vitality and **Sadness** optimism. However, when we are overcome with sadness and grief the Lungs are weakened. Because the Lungs govern the Ki, sadness 'dissolves' Ki and tiredness results. Moreover, it is now well known that prolonged depression weakens the immune system. This can be explained by the fact that the Lungs also govern the Defensive Ki.

THE EXTERNAL CAUSES OF DISEASE

Whereas the Internal Causes of Disease are relatively subtle and arise from within, the External Causes are of a physical nature and encroach upon the body from the environment. They are referred to as 'external pathogenic factors' and are climatic in origin. They include:

- Wind
- Cold
- Heat/Fire
- Summer-Heat
- Dryness
- Dampness

Susceptibility to these pathogenic factors depends both on the strength of their impact on the body, and the body's strength in resisting them. Living in a region of extreme weather conditions will make diseases of an External origin common. However, those with a poor constitution and weak Defensive Ki will fall prey to the same diseases in a similar but less extreme climatic region.

These climatic terms refer both to the origin of the symptoms and the type of symptoms that are manifesting. They are primarily used as a means of classifying disharmonies which are caused by the physical environment. All disharmonies of an External origin are Excess conditions. There may be an underlying deficiency of Ki which allows external pathogenic factors to penetrate, but they are Excess in nature because they must be dispelled before the body can recover.

Wind Whereas the other External causes of disease are more closely related to specific climatic influences, the term 'Wind' indicates a pattern of disharmony rather than a climatic factor. Wind is characterized by symptoms which in modern terms would be labelled as a cold or flu. At the onset of these symptoms, 'Wind' invades the body and penetrates to the Exterior level between the skin and muscles, where the Defensive Ki circulates. Because the Lungs are the most 'external' Organ of the body, and because they control the Defensive Ki, they are the first Organ to be affected by an invasion of Wind. Wind affects the dispersing and descending function of the Lungs, causing sneezing, blocked sinuses, muscular aching, headaches and an aversion to cold.

Wind is characterized by acute symptoms which reflect the action of wind in nature: it arises swiftly, changes quickly, and blows forcefully and sporadically. Climatic wind makes the trees shake and sway; pathogenic Wind causes shivering. Wind is Yang in nature and therefore tends to injure the Yin.

The presence of External Wind is indicated by a Floating pulse (see p.212), as the Ki rises to the superficial Defensive level of the body in order to fight off the pathogenic factor. There are two types of external wind: Wind-Cold and Wind-Heat.

Wind-Cold Wind-Cold is characterized by sneezing, shivering, an aversion to cold, cough, and a runny nose with white or clear mucous. There is also likely to be stiffness and aching (especially in the neck and back of the head), a light fever, and an absence of sweating or thirst. An invasion of Wind-Cold results in a pulse which is both Floating and Tight.

Wind-Heat is characterized by feverishness and sweating, thirst, cough, and nasal congestion with yellow mucus. A sore throat and headache are also likely to arise. In comparison to Wind-Cold, muscular aching and aversion to cold will be mild, whereas fever will be heavy. Wind-Heat results in a pulse which is both Floating and Rapid.

Cold External Cold may penetrate into the body of those people who live or work in cold conditions. It is also more likely among people who do not, or cannot, dress properly. Cold causes Ki-stagnation and results in contraction of the muscles and joints, cramping pain and watery discharges. It produces a Tight pulse (see p.214) and a pale tongue (see p.216).

Heat-Fire External Heat can penetrate the body of someone who lives or works in an excessively hot environment – in an overly hot kitchen or bakery, for example. However, Heat and Fire most commonly originate from the Interior. They combine with external pathogenic factors such as Wind or Damp to produce additional symptoms of a Hot nature.

Because of their strong Yang nature, Heat and Fire injure the Yin of the body. Apart from making one feel hot, Heat dries up the Body Fluids and causes thirst and a dry mouth. It can also cause burning pain.

Fire displays these same characteristics, but is stronger and more 'solid' than Heat. Fire more commonly dries out the stools or causes constipation, and can make the Blood 'boil over' to cause bleeding. It has a greater effect on the Mind and more often results in mental agitation and insomnia. Its tendency to move upwards means that it can produce mouth ulcers and a bitter taste in the mouth. Both Heat and Fire produce a Rapid pulse and a red tongue.

Summer-Heat Summer-Heat is a specific type of Heat invasion, only occurring as a result of exposure to very hot weather, as in the case of sunstroke. Like Heat and Fire, it damages the Yin of the body, causing thirst, sweating, headache, and dark and scanty urine. If Summer-Heat invades the Heart Protector it can cause delirium and possibly unconsciousness. It produces a Rapid pulse and a red tongue.

Dryness Dryness is another external pathogenic factor which attacks the moist Yin of the body. The extreme dryness of certain natural and artificial environments can lead to dryness of the mouth, the tongue, the lips and the throat. The stools may become dry and urination dark and scanty.

Dampness Dampness is heavy and cloying and so impedes the Yang of the body, especially the transformative function of the Spleen. Exposure to damp weather, wearing wet clothes and living in a damp environment may allow External Dampness to invade. External Dampness frequently penetrates the Channels and gathers in the joints to produce rheumatic symptoms. These are characterized by fixed dull aching, stiffness and swelling of the joints. External Dampness can also combine with Heat to generate a fever. The presence of External Dampness is indicated by a Full and Slippery pulse and a thick, sticky tongue coating.

Dampness can also be generated from within by a weakness in the function of the Spleen, involving the subsequent poor transformation and transportation of Body Fluids. This condition is often compounded by excessive consumption of Damp-producing foods such as dairy products and sugar. Internal Dampness is characterized by symptoms which arise much more slowly than External Dampness. It often causes tiredness and a heavy feeling in the limbs. It tends to sink to the Hara where it produces swelling and a sense of fullness. Internal Dampness collects in the chest to produce a feeling of congestion and commonly makes one feel heavy-headed. It is also evident in vaginal discharges and skin diseases involving pus. Internal Dampness may produce a Fine and Slippery pulse and a sticky tongue coating.

An important pathogenic factor which is similar to Dampness is Phlegm. Phlegm is also generated by an impairment of the body's ability to transform and transport Body Fluids. However, in the case of Phlegm production, this process involves not only the Spleen but the Kidneys and Lungs as well. Moreover, Phlegm is only produced internally, so is not an External cause of disease. Rather than sinking to the Hara, Phlegm tends to collect in the Stomach and rise to the Lungs, nose and throat. It can also 'mist the orifices' of the Heart and therefore cloud and confuse the Mind.

Both Dampness and Phlegm frequently combine with Heat and Cold, producing Damp-Cold and Damp-Heat, and Cold Phlegm and Hot Phlegm. Phlegm can also combine with Fire to form Phlegm-Fire. Dampness and Phlegm which are Cold in nature produce white or clear mucus and a white tongue coating; Damp-Heat, Hot Phlegm and Phlegm-Fire produce yellow mucus and a yellow tongue coating.

THE OTHER CAUSES OF DISEASE

The causes of disease which do not fit into the categories above are as follows:

- poor constitution
- poor dietary habits
- over-exertion
- excessive sexual activity
- trauma
- parasites and poisons

Poor Constitution

An individual's constitutional strength is dependent on the health of their parents, particularly at the time of conception. This is the moment at which the Pre-Heaven Essence is formed from the fusion of the parental Essences. The foetal Essence becomes dependent on nourishment from the Mother. Her health during the period of gestation is thus another important factor in determining the strength of the child's constitution.

One's inherited (or Pre-Heaven) Essence is largely, though not completely, predetermined. It may be prematurely drained through overwork, excessive sexual activity and drug abuse; or it can be preserved and enhanced through special ways of self-development. Traditionally these include Tai Ji Quan, Qi Gong and Taoist forms of meditation and breathing exercises. Through building up one's reserve of Qi, a person with a relatively weak constitution may supplement their Essence with additional strength.

Poor Dietary Habits

Diet is of course a major cause of ill-health and plays a role in the development of almost all diseases. The subject of diet and health is a huge one but we can take a brief look at its most important aspects.

Dietary patterns in the West have two main problems: the over-consumption of foods of an animal origin; and the excessive influence of technology on agriculture and food production. The heavy reliance on meat and dairy products leads to a diet which is overly rich in fats. In addition, the livestock which produces these foods are fed hormones and antibiotics in order to enhance their profitability. The encroachment of technology upon the modern diet is further apparent in the heavy use of chemical fertilizers and pesticides as well as the widespread presence of chemical additives in food. All these influences heighten the possibility of degenerative disease.

Malnutrition is another serious problem, both in the Third World and the poorer areas of the West. It seriously weakens the Ki and Blood and results in Spleen deficiency, making it harder to absorb and make use of the little nourishment which is taken. Over-eating also weakens the Spleen and Stomach, and leads to 'Retention of Food', characterized by a bloated feeling in the stomach, belching, nausea and gastric reflux ('heartburn').

Regularly eating foods which are excessively Hot or Cold in energy is also detrimental to health. Too many cooling foods (such as salads, fruit, fruit juice, and ice cream) can injure the Yang of the Spleen. This impairs its transformative function (a function which requires warmth) and so leads to the accumulation of Dampness and Phlegm. Abdominal swelling and diarrhoea commonly result.

Foods which are very Hot in nature include beef, pork, alcohol and spicy food. Eaten in excess, they can create symptoms of Heat in the Liver or Stomach. These include a burning pain in the stomach and a bitter taste in the mouth. Oily, fried and greasy foods will again lead to a build-up of Dampness and Phlegm, impairing in particular the function of the Spleen. Phlegm will be evident in congested sinuses and a thick tongue coating.

Generally speaking, it is considered that a healthy diet should include cereal grains and their products, vegetables, beans, fruits, seeds and nuts. Unless one is vegetarian, eating fish and white meat is preferable to the frequent consumption of red meat. Also advisable is the moderate use of cold-pressed oils (N.B. cold-pressed oils should not be used for cooking at high temperatures) and natural, unrefined sweeteners. Medicinal diets must always be based on an accurate assessment of the patient's needs.

Those who are predominantly Yang-deficient will require a greater degree of warming foods such as cereal grains and cooked vegetables in their diet. They will do well to make use of items such as ginger and garlic in their cooking, both of which strengthen the body's Yang functions. Those patients who are predominantly Yin-deficient will need a higher proportion of cooling and moistening foods, such as lightly-cooked or raw vegetables and fruit. Special foods to tonify the Yin include pumpkin and fruits in general.

Food should always be eaten in a calm and settled state. Eating when upset or worried, eating in a hurry, or eating and working at the same time will deplete the Stomach and Spleen and impair digestion.

Over-Exertion Mental and physical over-exertion is a frequent cause of health problems in the West. Adequate rest is always necessary to replenish one's reserve of Ki. Insufficient rest over a number of months or years will mean that the body will have to draw on the Essence for additional strength. This will ultimately lead to a depletion of the Essence and to a weakening of the constitution.

Physical overwork puts a particular strain on the Spleen because it dominates the muscles. Repetitive use of certain muscles may cause localized Ki or Blood stagnation. Shiatsu therapy can do much to alleviate these conditions because of the effect it has on promoting circulation and improving muscle tone. An associated form of physical over-exertion is to found in people who engage in irregular and exhausting exercise, thus injuring Ki. On the other hand, a lack of exercise will lead to stagnation of Ki.

Because the Spleen houses Thought, it is easily weakened by excessive mental activity. Mental overwork also tends to consume the Yin of the body and therefore depletes the Stomach and Kidneys.

Excessive sexual activity has in the East traditionally been viewed as depleting to one's vital energy. The sexual energies of both men and women are derived from the Kidney-Essence. The body draws on the Essence in order to achieve ejaculation and orgasm. When there is insufficient time allowed between sexual activity for the replenishment of the Essence, and it outstrips one's reserve, a deficiency of Essence will ensue.

Excessive Sexual Activity

What is considered excessive sexual activity therefore depends upon the strength of one's Essence. The Essence reaches a peak in the early twenties and then begins to decline slowly. It also varies according to the individual: because some people have a strong constitution, they can engage in a relatively greater degree of sexual activity without depleting their Essence.

There is also a distinction to be made between men and women. Male sexual energy is more closely related to the Essence than female sexual energy. Ejaculation for men therefore represents a greater loss of Essence than orgasm for women. However, women also lose Essence through the process of childbirth, and may become deficient when the birth of one child is too quickly followed by another.

Strengthening the sexual function and replenishing the Essence requires treatment of the Kidneys, the basis of these energies. Kidney-Yang is responsible for mobilizing the Essence, especially in men; a deficiency will lead to impotence and premature ejaculation. Kidney-Essence and Kidney-Yin are especially important for the nourishment of the Uterus; their deficiency may cause infertility.

Trauma refers to physical accidents such as broken bones and bruising. Traumas result in localized stagnation of Ki, and stagnation of Blood if they are serious. Occasionally they cause long-term stagnation of Ki or Blood, especially when combined with other causes of disease such as External Dampness. External factors more easily penetrate into areas of the body weakened by a previous trauma and complicate an existing problem.

Trauma

Parasites – in the form of worms – and poisons are causes of disease which most frequently affect children. Clearly, they are problems which are not easily treated through Shiatsu.

Parasites and Poisons

Chapter 10

The Five Elements

INTRODUCTION

The Five Elements – Water, Wood, Fire, Earth and Metal – are an important aspect of Traditional Oriental Medicine. As an energetic system calling for intuitive insight and logic, it provides the Shiatsu practitioner with a tool to understand their patient physically, psychologically and spiritually. There are a number of points to grasp about the Five Elements before exploring them in detail individually.

It is significant that the Five Elements consist of five energetic stages rather than four, as in the Western tradition of Fire, Earth, Air and Water. Esoteric philosophers have understood the number five to symbolize dynamic interchange, and thus to represent Nature. This is precisely how the Five Elements are best understood: as stages of transformation which interconnect on every level of the natural world and the human microcosm of the bodymind.

Seeing the Five Elements as phases of a process rather than fixed representations of matter is supported by the literal meaning of the Chinese term for the 'Five Phases': *wu xing*. *Wu* means 'five', and *xing* means 'walk' or 'move'. The Five Elements express the 'five movements' of the Universe. As emblems of Nature they relate to a multitude of phenomena (season, colour, emotion and so on), but express the energetic quality of those phenomena as if they were different 'movements' of a whole. From this viewpoint, the Five Elements can be seen as an extrapolation of the movements of Yin and Yang (see Fig. 10.1).

THE CREATION CYCLE

Let us look at how the Five Elements embody the energetic stages of Yin/Yang. The Water Element possesses the Yin quality of life at rest; energy which is in a floating state (as in Winter). Wood gives this potential state the Yang qualities of direction and growth; energy rising (as in Spring). Growth leads to self-awareness, central to the Fire Element; energy expanding and reaching a peak (as in Summer). Earth gives this awareness bodily form, balancing it with Yin; energy descending earthwards (as in Late Summer). Metal completes the cycle through exchanging the outworn for the new; energy gathering to be dispersed (as in Autumn). Metal is Yin in function because it acts as a stable meeting point. Each stage generates and is the 'Mother' of the next, its 'Child'.

Since the Five Phases theory was first systematized around 300 BC, this sequential order of the Elements, called the *Shen* or 'Creation' Cycle, underwent many changes, and may not in reality be fixed. The modern order outlined here, however, is logical. It is seen at work in Nature in the way that Water nourishes Wood; Wood burns to make Fire; the ashes of Fire decompose into Earth; Earth contains the ores of Metal; and Metal melts into 'Water' (the liquid state).

A SUMMARY OF THE ELEMENTS

The Water Element is associated with night-time and with rest. It provides us with the instinct for survival and the emotion of Fear, as well as the urge to procreate. It is the source of Will (*Zhi*) in the

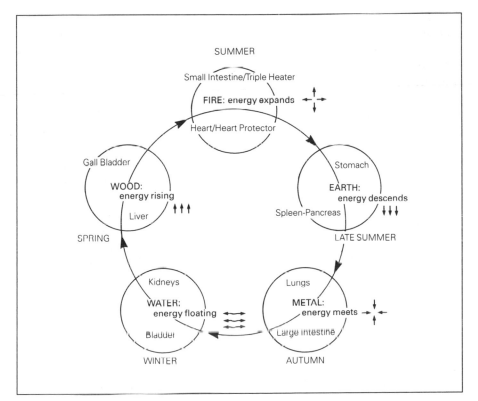

Fig. 10.1: Creation cycle

bodymind, and provides it with endurance. Water relates to the Yin (Zang) Organ of the Kidneys, which house the Essence (*Jing*), the basis of our constitutional strength. Its coupled Yang (Fu) Organ, also belonging to Water, is the Bladder. A person with a predominance of the Water Element will have a blue tinge to the colour of their face, a groaning sound in their voice, and a slight putrid odour (discernible near the chest or back). They may be slightly timid in character, or inwardly insecure.

The Wood Element is associated with the morning and with initiating action. It provides the ability to plan, control and assert, and affords the capacity for Anger. Wood relates to the Yin (Zang) Organ of the Liver, which houses the Ethereal Soul (*Hun*). The Ethereal Soul oversees our individual evolution, and is the source of hope and vision. The Yang (Fu) Organ which belongs to the Wood Element is the Gall Bladder, the seat of initiative. A person with a predominance of Wood energy will have a green tinge to the colour of their face, a slight shouting or clipped quality to the sound of their voice, and a faint rancid odour. They tend to be authoritative, well-organized and frequently irritable.

The Fire Element is associated with noon and activity at its peak. It represents our self-identity and urge to celebrate, bestowing the capacity for Joy and Love. Fire relates to the Yin Organ of the Heart, which houses the Mind (*Shen*). The Mind is the foundation of consciousness and the origin of thought and emotion. It is the most rarefied Ki of all. The Fire Element also encompasses the Organs of the Small Intestines, the Heart Protector and the Triple Heater. A person with a predominance of Fire energy will have a red tinge to the colour of their face, a laughing or tremulous quality to the sound of their voice, and a faint scorched odour. They are usually sensitive, excitable or emotionally changeable in nature.

The Earth Element is associated with the late afternoon and with a decrease in activity. It produces the ability to concentrate and analyse, granting the capacity for Pensiveness. Earth relates to the Yin Organ of the Spleen, which houses Thought (*Yi*). Thought provides the Mind with a logical process, just as the Spleen subjects food to a digestive process. Its coupled Yang Organ is the Stomach, the seat of our ability to listen and absorb. A person with a predominance of Earth energy will have a yellow tinge to the colour of their face, a singing quality to the sound of their voice, and a faintly sweet, or fragrant odour. They are often sympathetic listeners and have a tendency to worry.

The Metal Element is associated with the evening and a balance between activity and rest. It provides us with a sense of boundary across which we can take in and let go. Connected to the process of 'letting go' is the emotion of the Metal Element: that of Grief. Metal relates to the Yin Organ of the Lungs, which houses the Corporeal Soul (*P'o*). The Corporeal Soul gives us our 'animal' vitality and inherent optimism; when it is stricken we become despondent. The associated Yang Organ of the Metal Element is the Large Intestines. A person with a predominance of Metal energy will have a white tinge to the colour of their face, a subtle weeping quality to the sound of their voice, and a faint rotten odour. Although they can easily feel 'invaded', they quickly become melancholic if they 'lose touch' with those important to them.

A second set of relationships exist between alternate Elements of the Shen Cycle. In its normal clockwise movement, this interaction is known as the *Ko*, or 'Control', Cycle. The Ko Cycle may be expressed through the imagery of Nature as follows: Wood is cut by Metal; Metal is melted by Fire; Fire is extinguished by Water; Water is channelled by Earth; and Earth is penetrated by Wood (see Fig. 10.2).

The Control Cycle

To illustrate this 'control': the Water Element, through providing the 'Bone Marrow' that fills the brain, anchors the Mind of the Fire Element, whose underlying nature is to expand. The expansive radiance of the Self found in Fire controls Metal's tendency to concentrate and refine. Metal controls Wood through providing it with the sense of boundary and structure it needs to maintain order. The free-flow of energy in Wood ensures that Earth's transformative processes are smooth and harmoniously ordered. Finally, Earth harnesses the primordial power of Water by channelling it into physical processes.

The Shen and Ko cycles reflect two different 'movements' of the Five Elements. The Shen Cycle relationships are relatively more Yin: they are mutually nourishing and unifying. Ko Cycle interaction is relatively

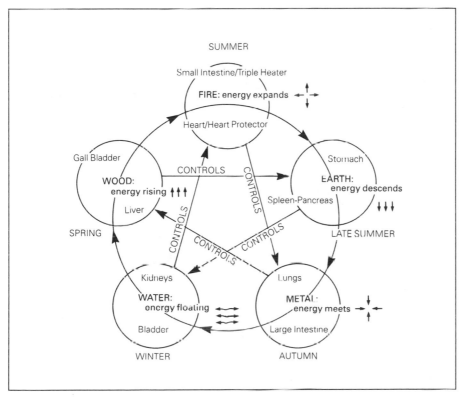

Fig. 10.2: Control cycle

more Yang: it reflects the antagonistic qualities of the Elements. Here they set mutual limits and so give each other structure, producing a cycle of 'control'.

THE FIVE ELEMENTS IN SHIATSU

The Five Elements serve the Shiatsu practitioner in three interconnected ways: they can enhance accurate physical diagnosis; provide a comprehensive model for understanding and treating the patient on an emotional level; and deepen philosophical insight.

On a level of physical diagnosis, they highlight the functions of the Organs they are associated with, making their dysfunctions clearer. They are not, however, an important means of understanding disease in Oriental Medicine, and are secondary to a thorough grasp of the Theory of the Organs (the *Zangfu*). It was only relatively recently in the history of Chinese Medicine, in the Song Dynasty (960–1279 AD), that the interactions of the Five Elements were commonly employed in the diagnosis and treatment of illness. Nevertheless, they provide a flexible yet revealing model for understanding the patient psychologically, and can lead the attentive practitioner to a deep insight into the Internal cause of a disease.

No one is in a state of perfect harmony: we all have certain psychological tendencies which, when over- or under-activated, concentrate emotional energy in certain Elements and not others. Each of the five basic 'attitudes' (or *zhi*) – Fear (Water), Anger (Wood), Joy (Fire), Pensiveness (Earth) and Grief (Metal) – are necessary to complete our character. But when we get 'stuck' in one or two of these 'attitudes' they can intensify into 'passions' (*qing*) and so dominate the psyche.

For example, we have seen from our observations of the Ko Cycle that the Water Element 'controls' Fire, partly through 'rooting' the mind. If the Water Element becomes afflicted, both physically and psychologically, through over-work and mental strain, the Kidneys (Water) will fail to provide a secure foundation for the Heart (Fire). This allows the Mind to become over-excited and nervous. When coupled with a vague sense of fear precipitated by a weakened Water Element, feelings of anxiety may result.

Understanding the causation of anxiety from this perspective allows the Shiatsu practitioner to formulate an appropriate and effective treatment strategy. In this particular case, they should consider tonifying the Channels and associated areas of the Kidneys, as well as dispersing those of the Heart. Particular emphasis could be given to treatment of the following Tsubos: Kidney-6 (tonifies Kidney Yin and calms the Mind); Bladder-23 (strengthens Ki of Kidneys); Directing Vessel-4 (supports firm foundation of the Kidneys and roots the Mind); Heart-7 and Directing Vessel-15 (both calm the Heart and the Mind).

The Five Elements are therefore of great practical value in Shiatsu.

They can, at the same time, be of spiritual value to the natural healer. As a dynamic model of wholeness, they can allow us to look at our own life and assess, in a non-judgemental spirit, the relative balance of its different parts. For example, we may ask ourselves how we touch our deepest core and self renew (Water)? Whether we have a harmonious sense of achievement in life, being neither driven nor without vision (Wood)? Can we allow ourselves to love, and so be essentially self-fulfilled (Fire)? Do we truly listen to life, integrate experience and allow it to change us (Earth)? Finally, do we feel 'connected' to others, neither cut-off or impinged upon (Metal)?

As a tool of meditation we can employ the Five Elements on a more subtle level through visualizing those Elements in which we may feel particularly challenged. For example, to cultivate self-confidence and easy authority (Wood), we may visualize the rooted sturdiness of a tree, its limbs of strength reaching upwards. To relieve melancholy and revive the brilliance of inner Ki (Metal), we can visualize the diamond or crystal and its vibrant power to receive, refract and radiate, simultaneously, always in the present moment.

Now we are ready to explore each of the Five Elements and their associated Organs in detail.

Chapter 11

Water: The Kidneys and Bladder

The natural point of departure for an in-depth discussion of the Five Elements and their associated Yin and Yang Organs begins with the Water Element. This is because Water is representative of life's beginning. As Lao Tzu says in the Tao Te Ching: 'Water gives life to the ten thousand things and does not strive.'

In the world's oldest creation myth, the ancient Sumerians ascribed the creative principle to the sea. The same hieroglyph also represented both the Goddess of Water and human sperm. To the Chinese, too, the Water Element symbolized the source of life, containing within itself life's many possible creations.

In the body, this originating aspect of the Water Element is reflected in the Original Ki and its substantial basis, the Essence (or *Jing*, both of which are controlled by the Kidneys. The Kidneys are the Yin Organ of the Water Element; the Bladder its Yang Organ. The Essence forms the 'core' of the bodymind and could be said, in scientific terms, to contain the genetic material needed for conception and new life.

The Source of Life provides the will-to-be and will-to-create: thus it is the Kidneys which house the Will (or *Zhi*) of the bodymind. The Will provides the instinct for survival and drive to procreate. It is when the Will is threatened in some way that fear emerges within the psyche. When the Will is strong we are invested with self-confidence and an innate trust in what life will bring. The energetic centre of the Will is located deep in the Hara, at the 'Gate of Vitality', the source of our strength and stability.

The season of Water is Winter, when the energy of the Earth is in a dormant, floating state, and when the potential plant is but a seed, waiting for the warmth of Spring. The nature of the Water Element may be further explored and more clearly understood through an analysis of the functions of its associated Yin organ, the Kidneys.

THE FUNCTIONS OF THE KIDNEYS

Store the Essence The first function of the Kidneys is to store the Essence which in turn governs the processes of birth, growth, reproduction and development. We have already looked at the Essence in some detail and have seen that it is closely related to the Kidneys. The Kidneys host and sustain the Essence, and together they ensure that we develop according to an original 'plan'. This plan is unique to each individual, and is contained in the genetic code formed at conception. It is the work of the Kidney Essence to sustain this plan against a variety of environmental and pathogenic influences. It thus ensures the integrity and cohesion of the individual.

The Essence manifests itself over time through the process of physical and mental growth. Problems relating to the Essence may result in retarded growth or premature aging. Because the Essence provides the basis for sexual development, infertility or a lack of sexual vitality can also occur.

A natural and harmonious decline is as much an expression of a healthy Essence as is normal growth and development in children. If one expresses one's willpower wisely, the Essence is well preserved and diminishes slowly. The wise person adapts to its decline and makes perfect use of the Essence they have, thus maintaining vitality.

Produce the Marrow

The second function of the Kidneys, closely related to the first, is that they 'produce the Marrow, fill up the brain and control the bones'. Just as they provide, through the Essence, the genetic structure of the body, so they provide it with physical structure in the form of the bones and teeth. However, the Oriental concept of the Marrow includes not only the bone-marrow, but the brain, nerves and spinal cord as well. The Marrow is part of the Essence and therefore fundamentally Yin in nature. Forming the physical basis of the nervous system it hosts its energetic Yang polarity, the Mind (or Shen).

Govern Water

The third main function of the Kidneys is directly associated with their Western physiological function; namely, that the Kidneys govern Water in the body. The Kidneys have a close relationship with the Lower Heater, which includes the entire lower abdomen below the level of the umbilicus. The organs in this area are often compared to a 'drainage ditch', as they are responsible for the excretion of impure Body Fluids. The Kidneys may be thought of as a 'gate' which opens and closes to control this flow of fluids. When Kidney-Yang is deficient, the gate is too open, leading to copious, clear urination. When Kidney-Yin is deficient, the gate is too closed, leading to scanty, dark urination.

Control the Reception of Ki

This function of the Kidneys highlights their close relationship with the Lungs. The Kidneys grasp and anchor the Ki descended by the Lungs following inhalation. If the Kidney-Yang becomes deficient, and this function weakens, Ki will become trapped in the chest and asthma may develop.

Open into the Ears The Kidneys open into the ears, because the ears depend upon sustenance from the Essence to function well. Problems related to hearing, such as tinnitus (ringing in the ears) may be related to Kidney weakness.

Manifest on the Hair Finally, the Kidneys manifest on the hair, which, like the ears, depends upon the Essence for normal growth. Abundant, shining hair reflects a vital Kidney-Essence; hair which is thin, brittle and greying may indicate that the Essence is weakening.

THE FUNCTIONS OF THE BLADDER

The role of the Bladder in 'The Yellow Emperor's Classic' is compared to that of 'a district official, it stores the fluids so that they can be excreted by its action of Ki transformation'. The function of the Bladder, therefore, is the transformation of fluids under the action of Ki supplied by the Kidney-Yang. It receives the impure fluids from the Small Intestines and transforms them into urine for storage and subsequent excretion.

SHIATSU TREATMENT OF THE KIDNEYS

In Shiatsu treatment, the Kidneys will often require tonification due to the key supportive role they play in relation to the other major Yin organs. First, the Kidney-Yin is vital for the nourishment of the Liver (Water feeds Wood). It also prevents the Liver from over-heating (due to the Liver's Yang nature and wide array of functions). The Kidney-Yang plays a crucial role in supporting the transformative action of the Spleen-Yang, providing it with the Fire necessary for digestion. The Heart relies on both the Kidney-Yang for force and the Kidney-Yin for nourishment; the Kidney-Yin also helps to anchor the Mind. Again, the Lungs rely on the Kidneys to 'grasp the Ki' derived from breathing. It is understandable, therefore, that the Kidneys are considered to be 'the root of Yin and Yang'.

Signs and symptoms common to Kidney problems in general include lower-back pain, dark rings under the eyes, a groaning sound in the voice, and feelings of insecurity, anxiety or fear.

Treatment of Kidney-Essence Deficiency In the Shiatsu clinic the most common type of patient requiring strengthening of the Essence is the elderly person with problems such as Osteoporosis, Osteoarthritis, loss of memory, loss of hair and teeth, and chronic fatigue. Because Ki and Blood deficiency are commonly involved, the tongue and face are likely to be a dull, pale colour, and the pulse Empty. The Kidney Channel will generally be Kyo in condition.

The practitioner should apply tonifying treatment to the Kidney Channel. The main Tsubos for tonifying the Essence are Kidney-3 and Directing Vessel-4. The Tsubo Bladder-23 (Kidney Yu Point) will support the Essence through strengthening the Kidneys. Tonification of Gall Bladder-39 is called for in cases of Osteoporosis, as it tonifies the Bone Marrow. The Tsubo Bladder-11 (Gathering Point for the Bones) also helps to strengthen the bones.

Treatment of Kidney-Yin Deficiency

It is important to remember that the Kidneys are the body's source of Yin (moisture, nourishment and cooling). Kidney-Yin deficiency is apparent when signs of Kidney weakness such as lower-back pain combine with those of deficient Yin. Signs of Yin deficiency include hot hands and feet, dry mouth and sweating at night, and dark, scanty urine. The pulse will be Empty at a deep level (see p.213). The tongue will be red and possibly cracked, peeled or without a coating (see p.215).

Fig. 11.1: Tonifying the two 'Sea of Ki' points

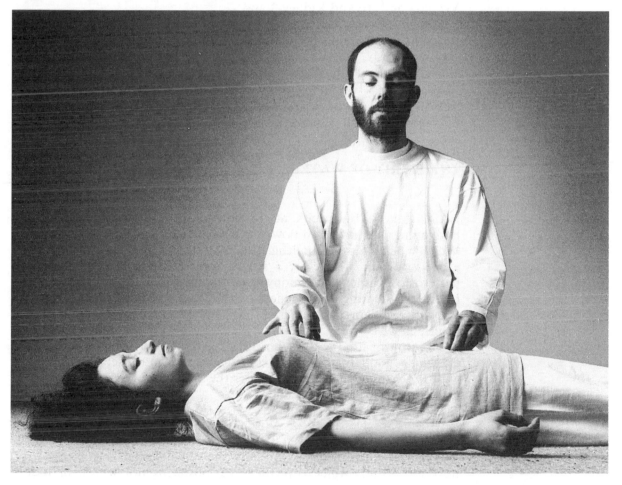

Kidney-Yin may be tonified through the sustained holding of the lower Hara and treatment of the Bladder Channel in the lower back. Tonify the Tsubos Kidney-6 and -3, Directing Vessel-4 and Spleen-6, all of which tonify Kidney-Yin.

(See Case Study Example No. 2 on p.225.)

Treatment of Kidney-Yang Deficiency

The Kidneys are closely related to the 'Gate of Vitality' and are the source of the body's Yang (i.e. warmth and motive force). A weakness of Kidney-Yang will directly affect the Yang of the entire body. Signs of Kidney-Yang deficiency include lethargy, pallor, coldness in the back and legs, weakness and oedema of the legs, loose stools and copious, clear urination. The pulse will be Empty and the tongue swollen and pale.

Kidney-Yang may be strengthened through the deep tonification of the lower Hara and treatment of the Bladder Channel in the lower back. Tsubos which strengthen Kidney-Yang include Bladder-23, Directing Vessel-4 and -6, and Kidney-3 and -7.

When weakness of Kidney-Yang leads to an impairment in the Kidney function of grasping the Ki, Lung-7 and Kidney-6 may be treated simultaneously. These two Tsubos in combination open the Directing Vessel, which, among other things, helps the Lungs and Kidneys to communicate. This may also be achieved by holding, with light finger pressure, both Directing Vessel-6 and -17, the lower and upper 'Sea of Ki' points (see Fig. 11.1).

THE SPIRIT OF WATER

Let us take a final look at the role of the Water Element in the bodymind. We have seen how Water is the source of our life-force and Will. When this is challenged and our survival is threatened we experience fear. However, a vague, subconscious fear may arise in patterns of Kidney disharmony, and manifest as insecurity, anxiety and mistrust. Treating the Kidneys with Shiatsu will help not only to alleviate problems such as lower-back pain, but will improve emotional health as well.

The tonification of Tsubo Bladder-52 ('Will Power Room') is especially good for restoring confidence and purpose. Tonifying the Kidney Channel in the chest restores the Will when there is timidity and a feeling of being overwhelmed.

According to Ted Kaptchuk,[1] the Water Element preserves the 'Virtue' (or 'Destiny') of Wisdom. It requires Wisdom to direct creatively the Will, as well as to harness and sustain it. It requires Wisdom, too, to cast aside fear when the Will is seriously challenged. To have an attitude which is neither over-powering nor wilful, or indeed easily overcome, ensures a wise and strong will-power.

This idea is crucial to good Shiatsu. The wise practitioner will work from their source, from their Hara. They will 'listen' to the patient's body and naturally find the right depth and strength of treatment. A strong and open Hara, one of the essentials of competent Shiatsu, is a sign of a healthy Water Element: they are ultimately one and the same.

The Water Element is also linked to technical ability – another essential ingredient of Shiatsu. The Kidneys are responsible for 'the power that is the underpinning of life from its beginning. This force or power is expressed with "skill" and "cleverness". with "know-how".'[2]

NOTES

1. Ted Kaptchuk, *The Way of the Spirit*, a public lecture held in London, November 1989.
2. Claude Larre, Jean Schatz and Elisabeth Rochat de la Vallee, *Survey of Traditional Chinese Medicine*, translated by Sarah Elizabeth Stang, Institut Ricci, Paris, and Traditional Acupuncture Institute, U.S.A., 1986, p.176.

Chapter 12

Wood: The Liver and Gall Bladder

As we have seen from our study of the Creation Cycle of the Five Elements, the raw force of Water yields to the organizing phase of Wood. The Wood Element does more than simply order and channel the drive of the Water Element, it lends it vision and gives it aspiration. Wood represents the 'giving of images'. Whereas Water is the seed, the symbol of potential growth, Wood is the shoot, and represents actual growth. The Wood Element is often called 'Tree-Phase', and encapsulates the rising energy of Spring-time.

The Yin Organ of the Wood Element, the Liver, is said in 'The Yellow Emperor's Classic' to be 'like an army's General from whom the strategy is derived'. The Liver harnesses the power of the bodymind and gives it a sense of direction. It ensures that our vital forces flow in harmony and according to plan. It is thus known as the 'Strategic Planner' among the twelve Organs, and is the source of our authority and decisiveness.

The Liver is assisted in this capacity by its paired Yang organ, the Gall Bladder, 'the upright Official that takes decisions'. The role of the Gall Bladder as 'decision-maker' is derived from its 'courageous' nature. The Gall Bladder takes the drive inherent in the Water Element and gives it decisiveness and action. It thus contributes to our courage and initiative.

The role of the Gall Bladder contrasts with the decision-making ability of the Small Intestines, which is based on its analytical power to 'separate the pure from the impure'. Rather than being a source of decisiveness as such, the Small Intestines help determine our clarity of mind.

THE FUNCTIONS OF THE LIVER

Smoothes the Flow of Ki The channelling action of the Wood Element is seen at work in the Liver's function of ensuring the smooth flow of Ki. This function is of vital importance to every area of the bodymind. If it fails, the mind becomes tense and bodily processes obstructed.

The stagnation and build-up of Ki are closely associated with frustration or depression. These emotions can both cause and result from Ki stagnation. We are more likely to get frustrated or depressed when the plans and visions of the Wood Element are thwarted. Getting angry also reflects a blockage of Ki, and sometimes helps release it. Anger which turns inwards appears in muted forms such as brooding resentment or deep depression. Longstanding emotions of a repressed nature can also generate Fire in the body.

Digestive problems are frequently caused by Ki stagnation due to Liver disharmony. These involve an array of symptoms reflecting a disruption of normal energy flow in the Stomach and Spleen. In terms of the Five Elements, Wood 'invades' Earth along the Control Cycle. The symptoms include indigestion, nausea, bloating, flatulence and sometimes epigastric pain.

The normal direction of Stomach-Ki is downwards: when this is disrupted there are signs of so called 'rebellious Ki'; energy moves upwards in the form of belching, gastric reflux ('heartburn') and vomiting. The normal direction of Spleen-Ki is upwards: when this is obstructed there are loose stools, diarrhoea and possibly prolapse.

Stagnant Liver-Ki can also obstruct the flow of bile, leading to poor digestion of fats, and in some cases jaundice. Feelings of tightness or oppression in the chest, of a lump in the throat and of distension of the breasts frequently reflect stagnation of Liver-Ki. Constipation may also have its root in this problem. General signs of stagnant Liver-Ki include a Wiry pulse, a purple tongue, rigidity of movement and chronic stiffness.

Stores the Blood

The second major function of the Liver is that it stores the Blood. This function seems simple in nature but effects the body in a number of ways. The Liver regulates the amount of Blood in circulation in accordance with levels of physical activity. During rest a large proportion of Blood flows to the Liver to be stored; when the body is active again, it returns to general circulation. This function ensures that the body receives adequate amounts of nourishment and energy.

If it becomes impaired and the Liver fails to store the Blood properly, Blood Deficiency may develop, producing such signs as fatigue, pallor, dizziness, dry skin, brittle nails and 'floaters' (spots) in the field of vision. The pulse will be Choppy or Thready and the tongue dull-pale and dry.

Controls the Sinews

The third function of the Liver is that it controls the sinews, i.e. the tendons, the ligaments and muscular action. Properly nourished by the Liver-Blood, the sinews will contract and relax in a way that ensures the smooth movement of the joints and ease of muscular action. When Liver-Blood is deficient, the tendons are more likely to become stiff, causing joint immobility and weakness in the limbs. More serious Liver disharmonies may lead to tetany and tremors involving the tendons.

Manifests in the Nails The nails depend, like the sinews with which they are associated, on the nourishment of Liver-Blood. Signs of deficiency of Liver-Blood include nails which have become indented, cracked and dry.

Opens into the Eyes Liver-Blood nourishes and maintains the eyes. Liver-Blood that is deficient may lead to dry and gritty eyes, poor vision and the presence of spots or 'floaters'. When there is excess Heat in the Liver the eyes often feel burning or painful. It should be remembered, however, that many of the Organs influence the condition of the eyes, so that not all eye problems are caused by the Liver.

The Liver Yu point, Bladder-18, may be treated for all eye problems. The Tsubo Gall-Bladder-37 (named 'Brightness') 'brightens the eyes'. Kidney-6 benefits the vision through nourishing the eyes.

THE FUNCTIONS OF THE GALL BLADDER

The functions of the Gall Bladder are relatively few and simple. We have already seen how the Gall Bladder plays an important role in decision-making and initiative. A person who pushes themself too hard will put particular strain on their Gall Bladder.

Its main physical function is the same as that of Western Medicine, the storage and excretion of bile. The efficiency with which this function operates is again dependent on the smooth flow of Ki. In turn, the health of the Gall Bladder influences the Liver's ability to regulate the Ki. The condition of these paired Organs is always closely connected.

SHIATSU TREATMENT OF THE LIVER AND GALL BLADDER

Treatment of Stagnant Liver/Gall Bladder Ki Stagnant Ki requires moving (i.e. dispersing): because to over-tonify the body of a person with stagnant Ki may exacerbate their condition. Happily, it is difficult to over-tonify with Shiatsu; it is more easily done with Acupuncture or Herbal Medicine.

When there is Ki stagnation, the Liver and Gall Bladder Channels will commonly present as Jitsu in condition. The Liver may also cause Ki stagnation in other Organs, especially the Stomach, Spleen, Heart, Heart Protector and Large Intestines, producing a Jitsu condition in these Channels as well. A variety of stretching techniques should be employed to move the Ki, with emphasis on opening the Gall Bladder Channel in the Side Position.

The main Tsubos to treat for stagnant Ki are Gall Bladder-34 and

Liver-3. Both Tsubos are called for when stagnant Liver-Ki affects the epigastrium and abdomen, causing problems such as nausea, indigestion and abdominal distension and pain. Gall Bladder-34 is especially important to treat in most cases of constipation. Both Tsubos should also be treated when there are muscular cramps and spasms in the body. Because Liver-3 has a strong calming action on the Liver, it is excellent for treatment of headaches.

Gall-Bladder-41 is another Tsubo which may be used for headaches due to stagnant Liver-Ki; it can also be dispersed to relieve breast pain and distension. The Tsubos Liver-13 and -14, both located under the rib cage, move the Liver-Ki when it disrupts the digestion. Both Tsubos help to harmonize Wood and Earth: Liver-13 is more effective for stagnant Liver-Ki 'invading' the Spleen; Liver-14 is more important for stagnant Liver-Ki 'invading' the Stomach. Among the many actions of the Tsubo Spleen-6 is its ability to smooth the Liver-Ki, especially in the Lower Heater. Finally, Heart Protector-6 is excellent for stagnant Ki in the chest, resulting in a sense of constriction or oppression.

Treatment of Liver-Blood Deficiency

Because the Liver stores the Blood, a deficiency of Blood will often create a Kyo condition of the Liver Channel, along with those of the Spleen and Kidney. It is important to tonify the Spleen and Kidneys as well as the Liver because of their central role in the formation of Blood. As the Yu Points have a powerful tonifying effect, treat Tsubos Bladder-18 (Liver Yu Point), Bladder-20 (Spleen Yu Point) and Bladder-23 (Kidney Yu Point). Applying moxibustion to the Yu Point of the Blood, Bladder-17, as well as Directing Vessel-4, will also strengthen Blood. Finally, tonifying Stomach-36 tonifies the Blood through increasing the digestive power.

Gynaecological Aspects of Liver-Blood

The Liver's function of storing Blood has a very strong relationship with both the normal and abnormal functioning of the female gynaecological system. If the Liver-Blood is deficient, it may well affect menstruation, causing amenorrhoea (a lack of periods). It is also possible for the Liver to transmit Heat into the Blood, making the Blood 'boil over' and cause menorrhagia (excessive menstrual bleeding) as well as metrorrhagia (bleeding between periods). The very close link between the Liver and menstruation also means that stagnant Liver-Ki often results in pre-menstrual tension and menstrual pain. The presence of dark clots in menstrual blood is a sign that Ki-Stagnation has led to Blood-Stagnation.

When periods are scanty or absent altogether in a woman with other signs of Blood Deficiency, treat them according to the same principles as those for Liver-Blood Deficiency (mentioned above), adding some sustained Hara work, especially where the abdomen is Kyo in condition.

In order to cool the Blood in cases of excessive menstruation or abnormal bleeding, one may disperse the Tsubos Liver-2 and Spleen-10.

The Liver Yu Point, Bladder-18, may be treated to regulate the Blood.

Bladder-18 is also called for when there is severe menstrual pain and the presence of clots due to Ki and Blood Stagnation. The Liver and Gall Bladder Channels in this instance will tend to be Jitsu in condition and should be dispersed. Disperse the Tsubos Gall Bladder-34, Liver-3 and Directing Vessel-6 to move Ki and Blood in the Hara.

Treatment of Liver-Yang Rising

In the Creation Cycle of the Five Elements, Water nourishes Wood. This can be seen at work in the fact that the Kidney-Yin moistens and nourishes the Liver. When a deficiency of Kidney-Yin leads to a depletion of Liver-Yin, the Yang of the Liver is allowed to predominate over the Yin. Unchecked by descending Yin, its natural tendency is to rise, causing symptoms which affect the head.

Headaches often occur, affecting the eyes and the sides of the head, the mouth and throat may become dry, and there may be dizziness and tinnitus (ringing in the ears). The patient may report a difficulty in sleeping and controlling their temper; they will often be irritable and angry. The pulse will be Wiry and the tongue red (especially along the sides). These symptoms may be coupled with those of Kidney-Yin deficiency, including lower back pain, night sweating and hot hands and feet.

It is common in this instance to find that the Liver and Gall Bladder Channels are Jitsu in condition and the Kidney Channel is Kyo. Disperse the Liver and Gall Bladder Channels and tonify that of the Kidney. In the case of frequent headaches, be sure to include techniques to release the neck and ease the shoulders and temporal areas of the head. The most important Tsubo to sedate Liver-Yang is Liver-3. Gall-Bladder-20 is called for in the case of frequent headaches and problems affecting the eyes. Triple Heater-5 may be dispersed in the case of headaches on the sides of the head. To strengthen Kidney-Yin, tonify the Tsubos Kidney-6 and -3, Directing Vessel-4 and Spleen-6.

(See Case Study Example No. 2 on p.225.)

Treatment of Liver-Fire

Fire in the Liver manifests most of the same signs and symptoms as Liver-Yang rising, but does not result from Kidney-Yin deficiency. Liver-Fire is an Excess pattern, whereas Liver-Yang rising is a pattern which involves both Empty and Excess conditions. Both patterns usually result from prolonged feelings of anger and frustration, although the emotions which generate Liver-Fire are either more extreme or repressed. Also, Liver-Fire is more often associated with the excessive intake of red meat, fatty foods and alcohol.

Liver-Fire can be distinguished from Liver-Yang rising in that it commonly produces a red face, red eyes, a bitter taste in the mouth and constipation. The pulse will be Full and Rapid; the tongue red with a yellow coating.

Liver-Fire will again tend to produce a Jitsu condition of the Liver and Gall Bladder Channels. Check the Heart and Heart Protector Channels as well; Fire is often transmitted from the Liver to the chest. Disperse the Liver and Gall Bladder Channels and the Tsubos Liver-2 and Gall Bladder-20, both of which sedate Liver-Fire.

Treatment of Liver-Wind

A deficiency of Liver-Blood or Liver-Yin, or a condition of extreme Liver-Heat, can on rare occasions give rise to a serious disharmony known as Internal Wind. Internal Wind should not be confused with External Wind: the two are fundamentally different. Internal Wind is generated by the Liver from within, and is characterized by dizziness and vertigo, tremor, rigidity, paralysis and convulsions.

Check whether the Liver Channel is Kyo or Jitsu in condition and treat accordingly. The main Tsubos to disperse Internal Wind are Liver-3, Gall Bladder-20 and Governing Vessel-16 and -20.

THE SPIRIT OF WOOD

A final, more subtle function of the Liver is that it houses the Ethereal Soul (or *Hun*). The Ethereal Soul is the part of the bodymind considered to survive after death and return to the world of immaterial existence. When properly rooted by the Yin and Blood, it provides us with our visionary capacity, which is intrinsic to the Wood Element; e.g. the Liver opens into the eyes.

If it becomes divorced from its physical 'home' the Ethereal Soul loses touch with its life's purpose and wanders aimlessly, divorced from reality. We lose our sense of living in the present. The bodymind compensates for this by erecting mental structures to mask a lack of inner meaning. But ultimately the rigidity which this encourages only creates frustration and intolerance. Ted Kaptchuk has indicated that the 'Virtue' of the Wood Element is Humankindness. Kindness and generosity renew our life with meaning; tolerance helps us to forgive those who have made us angry.

Among the essentials of competent Shiatsu, the Wood Element may be equated with continuity. An easy continuity from one technique to the next is a sign of the smooth flow of the practitioner's Ki. Their treatment plan should unfold effortlessly, ensuring that diverse techniques are linked together smoothly.

Chapter 13

Fire: The Heart, Heart Protector, Small Intestines and Triple Heater

The ascending energy of Wood culminates in the expansion of Fire. Its upward surge towards 'Heaven' leads it to the mind (or Shen) of the Fire Element, to the Self. Growth leads to wholeness, which is symbolized by the image of Fire: Fire both radiates from a central point and embraces its periphery with light. It evokes the formless dance of consciousness, and shines forth as Divine Ruler of the bodymind.

Joy and love are the principle emotions ascribed to the Fire Element because they are the natural expressions of pure Being, the basic ground of awareness. Whereas the Will emerges from below and the Soul reaches upwards, the Mind occupies the central residence of the Heart. It is emotional in nature because all feelings, including those of the other Elements, pour through it.

The season of Fire is Summer, when the life processes of Nature reach a high point of activity, and the Yang energy of the Sun is at its peak.

THE FUNCTIONS OF THE HEART

Of the four Organs within the Fire Element, the Heart is the most important. Its two primary functions are to govern the Blood and blood vessels and to house the Mind.

Governs the Blood The Heart governs the Blood in a way that is similar to its function in Western Medicine: it acts as a pump which circulates blood around the body. However, Oriental Medicine also states that the Heart is the site for the final stage of Blood production. According to Oriental Medicine it is in the Heart where the transformation of Food-Ki into Blood takes place. The Heart and the Blood are closely interdependent: the Heart ensures the Blood's vitality through its proper circulation, and the Blood in turn nourishes the Heart and helps it to anchor the Mind. Together they help determine the constitutional strength of an individual.

When the Ki or Blood of the Heart are weak, the circulation may be sluggish and the extremities cold. The person will feel tired and unenthusiastic.

A central function of the Heart unique to Oriental Medicine is that it houses the Mind (or Shen). There are five main aspects to the Mind, those of: basic consciousness; mental activity (including the emotional); thinking; memory; and sleep. When the Heart is in good health and properly nourished by the Blood, consciousness is clear and the thinking process normal. There will be a well-balanced emotional life, a strong memory and restful sleep. Because they nourish the Heart both the Blood and the Yin help to anchor the Mind and thus keep it calm and peaceful. A Mind which is harmonious is said to be discerned in eyes through which its brilliant sparkle shines. **Houses the Mind**

When the Heart is undernourished by the Blood and Yin, the Mind becomes 'ungrounded' and hyperactive. Feelings in general are intensified, and excessive 'Joy' manifests in the form of nervousness and excitement. The person will feel 'on edge', and will be more vulnerable to fright and shock, as their centre of consciousness will be less stable. A Mind which is seriously disturbed may result in behaviour which would be classified as 'manic' by Western Medicine.

An obviously milder and more common condition frequently involving the Fire Element is anxiety; a feeling of unease which includes a degree of both worry (Earth) and apprehension (Water) Again, the Mind cannot settle and occupy its residence within the Heart. Such distress may be compounded by a lack of Joy.

As part of its function of ruling the Blood, the Heart also controls the blood vessels. A healthy Heart will mean strong blood vessels and a clear, regular pulse. **Controls the Blood Vessels**

That the Heart manifests in the complexion demonstrates the link between a healthy circulation and a lustrous, rosy complexion. **Manifests in the Complexion**

The tongue is considered to be an extension of the Heart, and reflects in its shape and colour the condition of the Heart. Although the tongue shows the condition of all the Organs, it has particular bearing on that of the Heart. Heat in the Heart will often cause red, painful tongue ulcers as well as a bitter taste. The Heart also controls speech, and disharmonies occasionally lead to speech impediments such as stuttering. Heart problems may also mean that a person will talk incessantly or laugh without reason. **The Heart Opens Into the Tongue**

Because of the close relationship between the Blood and Body Fluids, **Controls Sweat** the Heart controls sweat. When the Heart-Ki is weak there may be spontaneous sweating; a lack of Heart-Yin often leads to sweating at night.

THE FUNCTIONS OF THE HEART PROTECTOR

Although the Heart Protector (or Pericardium) is paired with the Triple Heater, it is in reality closely related to the Heart. Forming the outer covering of the Heart, it protects it against external pathogenic invasion (mainly Heat). The Heart Protector will bear the brunt of any such attack in order to shield the Mind from danger. When such situations do occur they involve External Heat causing high fever and delirium.

The Heart Protector also aids the Heart in functions of governing the Blood and housing the Mind. The Tsubos of the Heart Protector Channel are as important as those of the Heart, and can be used to treat the same conditions. Psychologically, the condition of the Heart is indicative of one's relationship with one's Self, whereas that of the Heart Protector reflects the way we relate to others. Treatment of the Heart Protector Channel is often appropriate for people experiencing distress in relationships.

THE FUNCTIONS OF THE SMALL INTESTINES

The function of the Small Intestines is to separate pure from impure food and fluids. It receives food and drink which has been 'rotted and ripened' by the Stomach, and continues the process of transformation by separating the 'clean' part for distribution by the Spleen. The 'dirty' part is transported to the Large Intestines for its excretion in the form of stools, and to the Bladder to be eliminated as urine. The Small Intestines' function of discrimination extends to the mental sphere in the form of decision-making. In this way it has an influence on the clarity of the Mind's thought processes.

Disharmonies of the Small Intestines are closely related to those of the Spleen, as both organs are central to the transformation of nourishment.

THE FUNCTIONS OF THE TRIPLE HEATER

The Triple Heater is the only 'Organ' which does not possess a precise physical form in the same way as the other twelve Officials. It comprises Three 'Heaters' (or 'Burners'): the Upper Heater occupies the thorax; the Middle Heater the space between the diaphragm and the navel; and the Lower Heater the area below the navel.

Each Heater produces Body Fluids with a different form and function: the Upper Heater can be compared to a 'mist', distributing fluids throughout the body as a 'vapour'; the Middle Heater is likened to a 'bubbling cauldron', the site of digestion and the transportation of nutrients; and the Lower Heater is like a 'drainage ditch', from which fluids are separated and excreted. It is the work of the Triple Heater as an Organ to ensure the free passage of Body Fluids between these three regions, and to help regulate their distinctive functions. Thus, according to 'The Yellow Emperor's Classic': 'The Triple Heater is the Official in charge of irrigation and the control of the water passages.'

The breadth of the Triple Heater's function is due to its intimate connection with the Gate of Vitality (*Ming Men*), located between the Kidneys at the Tsubo Governor Vessel-4. It is the Triple Heater which directs the Original Ki (the Ki derived from the Essence) from the Gate of Vitality to every Organ and Channel of the body. The Triple Heater thereby helps to warm the Organs, sustain the Heart and energize the brain – all through distributing the Original Ki generated in the Hara. By extending the Original Ki to the body's periphery, the Triple Heater furthermore contributes to the strength of the Defensive Ki, thus helping to protect the body.

A secondary aspect of its warming and protecting function is its role in supporting the fascia which insulate the organs, i.e. the pleura, peritoneum and diaphragm.

The Triple Heater Channel should always be treated whenever there is a lack of strength in the Hara. It can be used to both support the Original Ki and move Ki in the entire body. This latter function makes it useful whenever stagnant Ki accumulates, especially in the Liver, Stomach and Large Intestines. The Triple Heater Channel may be treated in cases of chronic debility, coldness, constipation, parietal headache and ear infection.

SHIATSU TREATMENT OF THE HEART AND HEART PROTECTOR

The Heart and Heart Protector are of great importance in Shiatsu for the role they can play in the treatment of mental and emotional problems. A general sign of Heart distress is seen in the patient who is anxious and complains of palpitations. The exact nature of the condition is revealed by other signs and symptoms.

Deficiency of Heart-Ki manifests as tiredness, pallor, sweating, palpitations and shortness of breath on exertion. There may well be anxiety and sadness. The pulse will be Empty and the tongue pale.

Treatment of Heart-Ki Deficiency

It is clearly necessary in this case to administer Shiatsu which is tonifying in nature, concentrating on the Kyo Heart and Heart Protector Channels. Check whether the Kidney and Spleen Meridians are not also Kyo.

The main Tsubos to tonify Heart-Ki are Heart-5, Pericardium-6, Bladder-15 (the Heart Yu Point), and Directing Vessel-17 (which strengthens the Ki of the chest). Directing Vessel-6 should be tonified to raise the Ki of the whole body.

Treatment of Heart-Blood Deficiency

Deficiency of Blood affecting the Heart presents itself with symptoms which include palpitations, dizziness and a dull, pale complexion. The Blood's failure in helping the Heart to house the Mind leads to a poor memory, insomnia, and troubled, dream-filled sleep. It also means that the patient is likely to be anxious and easily startled. They will sometimes feel unable to cope with their responsibilities. The pulse will be Thready or Choppy; the tongue will be dry and a dull pale colour.

Treatment of Heart-Blood again calls for tonification of the Kyo Heart and Heart Protector Channels. The Spleen, responsible for the production of Blood, is also likely to exhibit a Kyo condition.

The Tsubo Heart-7 should be tonified as it nourishes the Blood and calms the Mind. Heart-Blood may also be strengthened through the treatment of Directing Vessel-15, excellent for allaying deep anxiety. Important Tsubos for the tonification of Blood in general include Bladder-17 (Yu Point of the Blood), Bladder-20 (Yu Point of the Spleen) and Directing Vessel-4.

Treatment of Heart-Yin Deficiency

This pattern presents itself as an array of symptoms which combine those of deficient Yin with those of a troubled Heart. The condition is similar to that of deficient Heart-Blood, as in both cases the Mind becomes agitated, deprived of its 'home'.

Symptoms of Heart-Yin deficiency include palpitations, anxiety and restlessness, There will again be a failing memory, insomnia and sleep which is disturbed by dreams. However, there will also be the typical Yin deficient signs of feeling hot or slightly feverish, of sweating at night, and of thirst and a dry mouth. Also, the patient may have red cheeks, and hot hands and feet.

In this condition, the Heart and Heart Protector Channels should be Kyo and in need of tonification. (If they are Jitsu, the condition is likely to be a Full one such as Heart-Fire.) Heart-Yin Deficiency also requires the tonification of Kidney-Yin, upon which it relies for nourishment.

Heart-6 is the main Tsubo along the Heart Channel to tonify the Heart-Yin. Directing Vessel-15 will strengthen the Heart and dispel anxiety and restlessness. Spleen-6 and Kidney-6 are important to tonify the Yin in general, as well as to calm the Mind. Finally, Directing Vessel-4 anchors the Mind through nourishing the Yin and Blood.

So far we have looked at Deficient patterns of Heart disharmony, all of which require tonifying Shiatsu treatment. If, however, symptoms involving the Heart are found on a person whose Heart Channel is clearly Jitsu, their condition is likely to be Full in nature. There could be Fire, excessive Phlegm or Stagnation of Blood in the Heart. Such problems are often more acute than those of an Empty nature, and should be approached with caution, calling for a gently dispersing style of treatment.

Treatment of Full Heart Conditions

Heart-Fire is distinguished by feelings of heat throughout the day and night, by a red face, a bitter taste in the mouth, tongue ulcers and blood in the urine. There is usually a significant degree of mental agitation, occasionally combined with excessively extrovert or manic behaviour. Insomnia is also common. The pulse will be Rapid and Full; the tongue will be red (especially at the tip) and have a yellow coating. The Heart and Heart Protector Channels will almost certainly be Jitsu in condition. Dispersal of the Tsubos Heart-8 and -9 are called for, as they both clear Heart-Fire.

Heart-Fire Blazing

When Phlegm 'mists the orifices' of the Heart, there is often severe mental disturbance and confusion, as the Mind becomes seriously clouded and loses touch with reality. The pulse will be Rapid, Full and Slippery and the tongue red with a thick yellow coating. The Heart and Heart Protector Channels will most likely be Jitsu in condition. Check the Spleen Channel for a Kyo condition, as Spleen deficiency will contribute to the production of Phlegm. Heart Protector-5 is the main Tsubo to clear Phlegm from the Heart and 'open the orifices', and should naturally be dispersed.

Phlegm in the Heart

Stagnant Heart-Blood is an advanced pathological condition of the Heart involving chest pain which often radiates down the left arm. The chest feels stuffy or constricted and the nails, lips and tongue may be purple or blue. The Heart, Heart Protector, Liver and Gall Bladder Channels are likely to be Jitsu in condition, and should be dispersed to move Blood in the chest. The main Tsubos for stagnation of Heart-Blood are Heart Protector-6 and Conception Vessel-17, both of which strengthen the Heart and promote the flow of Blood.

Stagnation of Heart-Blood

THE SPIRIT OF FIRE

The Heart is the 'Supreme Governor' of the bodymind, and was equated by the ancient Chinese with the role of Emperor. Its imperial position among the twelve main Organs is directly related to its function of housing the Shen. The Shen encompasses every aspect of human consciousness, uniting each emotional, mental and spiritual activity into a single whole. All the five Elements contribute to the creation of Selfhood: Water gives it drive; Wood, vision; Earth allows it form; and Metal, relationship. But it is Fire which *represents* this Selfhood and gives it its uniqueness and cohesion. 'The Shen are that by which a given being is unlike another; that which makes an individual an individual and more than merely a person.'[1]

The Fire Element presides over the bodymind as its 'Divine Ruler', granting it the capacity for enjoyment and love. It is Fire's responsibility to reconcile the instinctive with the rational, the emotional with the spiritual, and to maintain their delicate equilibrium. The power to harmonize these often conflicting activities requires a sense of perfection. This sense is linked to the 'Virtue' of the Fire Element, which, according to Ted Kaptchuk, is Propriety: a fine intuition for what is fit and proper.

To help restore equilibrium to the unsettled Shen of a recipient calls for Shiatsu which is truly effortless and non-judgemental. This requires an empty mind – one of the essentials of competent Shiatsu. An empty mind will allow us to work from the Heart. At one with the Hara, we are able to convey and awaken Ki; at one with the Heart, we can centre and harmonize the Shen.

NOTES

1. Claude Larre, Jean Schatz and Elisabeth Rochat de la Vallee, *Survey of Traditional Chinese Medicine*, translated by Sarah Elizabeth Stang (Institut Ricci, Paris, and Traditional Acupuncture Institute, 1986), p.192.

Chapter 14

Earth: The Spleen and Stomach

The Earth Element takes the basic consciousness of Fire and gives it form. It does this through the creation of concrete thought, and putting ideas into action. Water imbues life with impetus, Wood harnesses it; Fire crowns life with self-awareness and now Earth must give it focus. Each Element nourishes the next. The self-orientation of Fire compensates for the goal-orientation of Wood; similarly, Earth's concern with the real modifies Fire's emphasis on the ideal. The Earth Element thus allows the Mind a vehicle through which it can explore and express itself on a practical level.

The nature of the Earth Element is to consolidate and maintain. Among the Five Elements it is one which occupies the Centre, the position from which it can most effectively bind together and sustain the other four. In order to nurture the bodymind it must be capable of absorption. However, crucial to absorption is the power to take that which is 'other' and make it one's own. This is the process central to Earth: that of transformation.

Earth's transformative function is apparent on two main levels: that of the digestion of food and its final conversion into Blood; and that of the process of mental cognition and Thought (Yi). Earth absorbs the sensations and perceptions of the bodymind, breaks them down like the soil, and makes them part of the Mind. This gives credence to the sympathetic nature of Earth, as does its urge to nurture.

Only transformation which is efficient yields productive results. Overthinking, the 'emotion' of Earth, often means remaining stuck in repetitive cycles of thought. This prevents energy from descending towards the earth, towards the realm of action. When Thought cannot reach conclusions and transform into reality then worry and obsessiveness ensue. Giving sympathy to someone soothes and settles their thoughts and helps them find understanding.

The nurturing aspect of Earth is an important one and is clearly reflected in the functions of its associated Organs, the Stomach and Spleen. The Stomach is the ultimate source of the body's nourishment and the Spleen the origin of the Blood. Together they play the role of Mother Earth, providing the body with sustenance.

THE FUNCTIONS OF THE SPLEEN

The Spleen is the primary Zang Organ of the Earth Element, and includes the pancreas as part of its functional unit.

Governs Transformation and Transportation

The first function of the Spleen is the transformation of ingested food and drink into Food-Ki, and the transportation of nutrients to the other bodily viscera. Food-Ki provides the raw material for the manufacture of Ki and Blood. It is derived from the 'pure essence' of food and is directed upwards by the Spleen to the Lungs and Heart. It is in the chest that Food-Ki combines with the 'Ki of clean air' to form Gathering Ki, and in the Heart that it is converted into Blood.

The Spleen is the main Organ of digestion due to its central role of transformation and transportation, and is the source of bodily Ki and Blood. Its importance is highlighted by the fact that it is the foundation of 'Post-Heaven Essence' (see p.127). The Spleen is also responsible for the transformation, separation and transportation of fluids. The 'clear' Body Fluids go to the Lungs for dispersal around the body and the 'dirty' part enters the intestines for further refinement.

A healthy Spleen ensures that digestion and absorption are efficient and normal, that there is a good appetite, and that bowel movements are regular. If this process is disrupted, digestion will be upset and the appetite poor. There will be abdominal swelling, loose stools and the accumulation of excessive Body Fluids in the form of Dampness, Phlegm or oedema.

Controls the Blood

The Spleen is not only responsible for the origin of Blood through the transformation of food, but 'controls' the Blood by keeping it in the blood vessels. A breakdown of this function may lead to such problems as haemorrhage or excessive menstrual bleeding.

Controls the Muscles and the Four Limbs

Because the Spleen is the basis of nourishment and its transportation around the body, it plays a major role in ensuring muscular strength, and thus 'controls' the muscles and the four limbs.

Opens into the Mouth and Manifests in the Lips

The action of chewing is the first stage in the transformation of food, and for this reason is closely connected to the Spleen. The Spleen, therefore, opens into the mouth and manifests in the lips. The Spleen produces the sense of taste as well as a feeling of appetite. Spleen dysfunction will manifest in either dry, cracked lips, indicating the presence of Heat, or pale lips, showing that Spleen-Ki is weak.

In addition to raising Food-Ki to the chest, the Spleen has the function of controlling the raising of Ki in a general sense. It 'lifts' the internal organs and so holds them in their proper place. Failure of this function leads to prolapse or herniation. **Controls the Raising of Ki**

Finally, the Spleen houses 'Thought', dominating the processes of thinking, analysing, concentrating and studying. In health, the Spleen ensures strong powers of reasoning and memory. When there is a deficiency of Spleen-Ki, the thought process will be unclear and the concentration cloudy. Such a person may have to expend a lot of mental energy in finding solutions, resulting in Overthinking and a further depletion of Spleen-Ki. **Houses Thought (Yi)**

THE FUNCTIONS OF THE STOMACH

The Stomach is perhaps the most important Yang Organ, forming, in conjunction with the Spleen, the 'Root of Post-Heaven Ki'. Pre-Heaven Ki, assimilated before birth by the Kidneys, is the source of our consitutional strength, whereas Post-Heaven Ki is formed after birth by the Stomach and Spleen from food and drink. Both the Earth Organs have a major influence on the quality of Ki and Blood.

The primary function of the Stomach is to control the 'rotting and ripening' of food. Through a process akin to fermentation, food is prepared by the Stomach for its refinement by the Spleen and its separation by the Small Intestines. Representing the first stage in the digestive process, it forms the very basis of bodily nourishment. **Controls the Rotting and Ripening of Food**

Along with the Spleen, the Stomach also controls the transportation of food essences to the entire body, particularly the muscles and limbs. If the Stomach-Ki is weak, the legs and arms will feel heavy and the person will easily tire. **Controls the Transportation of Food Essences**

The Stomach is said to control the descending of Ki by virtue of its action in sending down food to the Small Intestines. Whereas Spleen-Ki ascends and controls the raising of Ki, Stomach-Ki should descend. Failure of this Stomach function, often because of its disruption by Liver-Ki Stagnation, will lead to bloating, belching, gastric reflux, hiccup and vomiting – all signs of Stomach-Ki 'rebelling' upward. **Controls the Descending of Ki**

SHIATSU TREATMENT OF THE SPLEEN AND STOMACH

Spleen and Stomach Deficiency

A deficiency of Spleen-Ki produces a host of symptoms centring around weakness in the digestive processes and a resulting lack of available energy. Besides a dragging feeling of tiredness and weakness in the limbs, there is abdominal swelling, a lack of appetite, loose stools and a pale complexion. Spleen-Ki deficiency produces an Empty pulse and a tongue which may be pale and swollen.

Dampness and Phlegm may also accumulate due to an impaired transformation function. This is evident in fluid retention, feelings of heaviness and respiratory congestion. Dampness and Phlegm produce a Slippery pulse and tongue with a thick and sticky coating. In the case of Spleen-Yang deficiency, we can add to these symptoms feelings of cold, especially in the limbs. The pulse will be Deep and Weak and the tongue pale, swollen and wet.

A deficiency of Stomach-Ki will manifest the same symptoms, but with a greater emphasis on discomfort in the epigastric area. The pulse will be Empty and the tongue pale. When the Spleen and Stomach are deficient, their Channels will usually be Kyo in condition. The diagnostic area for the Spleen on the Hara (around the navel) will often be swollen or puffy and feel Empty to the touch.

The treatment of these deficient Spleen and Stomach patterns may be approached in basically the same way. In both cases tonify the Spleen and Stomach Channels, including the Tsubos Spleen-6 and Stomach-36. Treat the Tsubos Directing Vessel-12 (Bo point for the Stomach and Middle Heater) and Bladder-20 and -21 (Spleen and Stomach Yu Points). All these Tsubos have a strong tonifying action, especially when there are signs of Cold.

Excessive Dampness, especially when it has invaded the Spleen itself, may produce a Jitsu condition in the Spleen and Stomach Channels. Dispersing the Spleen and Stomach Channels as well as the Tsubo Stomach-40 will help clear Dampness and Phlegm.

The Spleen Channel is often Kyo in condition when there is Blood deficiency, evident in signs of dizziness, tiredness, dry skin, cracked nails and impaired vision. It is important in this case to tonify both the Spleen and Stomach Channels and so strengthen the digestion. It may also be necessary to tonify the Liver and Heart Channels, because these Organs are easily affected by Blood deficiency.

Retention of Food in the Stomach

When the Stomach-Ki stagnates, often due to Liver-Ki stagnation, a 'stuck' condition manifests and causes a sensation of abdominal fullness and bloating. Food is not properly digested and is 'retained' in the Stomach, leading to appetite loss, nausea and signs of Stomach-Ki 'rebelling' upwards, i.e. belching, acid regurgitation and vomiting. The pulse will be Full and Slippery or Wiry; the tongue will have a thick coating.

The Stomach Channel is usually Jitsu in this condition. Tsubos which relieve the Retention of Food and encourage Stomach-Ki to descend include Stomach-21 and Stomach-44.

Stomach-Yin Deficiency

The Stomach is said to be the origin of fluids in the body, and unlike the Spleen, can become deficient in Yin. This will produce symptoms of dryness, including a dry mouth and throat, thirst, and dry stools which lead to constipation. These problems will be coupled with epigastric pain and appetite loss. The pulse will be Floating, and the tongue red and possibly peeled or cracked in the centre.

The Stomach Channel is very likely to be Kyo in condition. Check the Kidney Channel also, as the Kidneys will be involved in any Yin-deficient pattern. Specific Tsubos to tonify are Stomach-36, Spleen-6 and Directing Vessel-12.

Phlegm-Fire in the Stomach

When Phlegm and Fire build up in the Stomach due to poor dietary habits, a Full condition ensues. Stomach Phlegm-Fire is characterized by feelings of burning and pain in the Stomach area, by constant hunger, bleeding gums, constipation, nausea and bad breath. There is often a strong desire to drink cold liquids in order to quell the Fire. Mentally, insomnia and worry are common. The more that Phlegm is involved, the greater the sense of congestion and disorientation. The pulse will be Rapid and Full due to Heat and possibly Slippery due to Phlegm. The tongue will be red with a thick, yellow coating.

Check the Stomach Channel: it is likely to be Jitsu and in need of dispersal. Disperse the Tsubos Stomach-21 and Stomach-44, both of which clear Heat from the Stomach. Disperse Stomach-40 to clear Phlegm.

THE SPIRIT OF EARTH

As thinking precedes physical action, it seems appropriate that Thought should be associated with the Earth Element. Thought is the first stage in the process of actualization, i.e. bringing ideas into reality. The higher purpose of Thought, and the 'Virtue' of the Earth Element,[3] is to explore the creative possibilities of the Mind.

Creativity is an alchemical process; taking the base metals of the Mind and converting them into the gold of art and philosophy. True art requires a sense of proportion and harmony – something which Thought derives from the Propriety of the Shen. At the same time, creativity releases us from the strictures of Propriety, and encourages us to explore the realm of the possible.

Creativity in Shiatsu is akin to fluency, an essential aspect of competent treatment. Fluency is the ability to draw on a wide variety of techniques in direct response to the recipient's needs. All techniques, however, should be based on the stable ground of support, another keynote of Earth.

Chapter 15

Metal: The Lungs and Large Intestines

Once the Earth Element has established consciousness on a physical plane it is left to Metal to complete the making of the Self by lending it boundary. Paradoxically, having a surface – a skin – allows us to interact with others and the environment; it provides us with a transmission point across which we can 'take in' and 'let go'.

The Metal Element is symbolic of our constant partaking of life, and is seen at work in the breath. It says, 'We are what passes through us,' and defines the Self according to its interaction with the external world. The more that we can 'open up' to our environment and at the same time relinquish the things of the past, the more vital and alive we are. This vitality is a manifestation of the Corporeal Soul or P'o, closely linked to the Lungs and the Metal Element in general.

Whereas the Ethereal Soul is future-orientated, the bodily or Corporeal Soul is concerned only with the present. The Corporeal Soul may be compared to the vibrant, ever-fresh world of young children, ceaselessly immersed in the exploration of the things around them.

Thus, when we lose someone or something dear to us, it is this very capacity – to be always in the moment – which loses hold. Our minds centre for a while on the past, as we go through a special process called Grief. It is only through grieving that we can learn a deeper acceptance of life and death, and therefore regain the present.

If, however, we never fully grieve, we are likely to remain 'stuck' in an acute awareness of what we have lost, and become melancholic and remorseful. The boundary between us and present reality will grow, and others will feel that we are 'out of reach' in some way. Such a person becomes dominated by the Metal Element because they cannot learn the process which is central to it: that of accepting and 'letting go'.

THE FUNCTIONS OF THE LUNGS

The functions of the Lungs are directly related to the process of respiration, and indirectly to the Heart and circulation.

Govern Ki and Respiration

When the Lungs inhale air they are extracting 'pure Ki' from their environment. Exhalation is a way of discharging 'dirty Ki'. Respiration thus ensures the continual renewal and freshness of bodily Ki.

The Lungs also dominate the formation of Ki in the chest. Food-Ki, made from refined food and drink, is directed by the Spleen up to the chest, where it combines with the 'pure Ki' of air to form Gathering Ki or 'Ki of the chest'. Gathering Ki forms the basis of Nutritive and Defensive Ki, and lends force to Lung and Heart function. A deficiency of Lung-Ki will directly affect the Ki of the whole body.

Control the Channels and Blood Vessels

Because the Lungs govern the Ki and Ki propels the Heart and circulation, the Lungs are said to control both the Channels and blood vessels. The Lungs are the most important Organ in the formation of Nutritive Ki, the Ki which flows not only in the Channels, but in the blood vessels as well. The circulation of Ki and Blood are closely connected, as the Blood relies on the Ki for its propulsion around the body. They are both greatly influenced by the strength of the Lung-Ki.

Control Dispersing and Descending

This important Lung function is associated with the Lungs' control of the Ki. The Lungs control the dispersing of both Defensive Ki and Body Fluids around the periphery of the body – to the space between the muscles and skin. When the Defensive Ki is spread evenly under the body surface it fulfils the role of protecting the body from pathogenic factors such as Cold and Dampness. It also warms the skin and muscles. Impairment of this function will cause a weakening of Defensive Ki and pave the way for invasion of the body by pathogenic factors, causing ailments such as colds and influenza.

The dispersal of Body Fluids by the Lungs ensures that sufficient moisture reaches the skin and muscles. The Body Fluids are distributed in the form of a 'fine mist'. (This is the form in which they appear in the region of the Upper Heater.) The Lungs also regulate the opening and closing of the pores on the skin surface. They ensure that perspiration is normal, i.e. neither excessive or deficient.

The Lungs have an important descending function. As they are the uppermost Organ of the body, it is important that their energy descends in order for Ki to 'communicate' with the rest of the body. The Lungs therefore have an important relationship with the Kidneys. The Lungs send Ki downwards and the Kidneys 'grasp' it. The Lungs also descend and provide Ki for the functioning of the Bladder and Large Intestines. This descending function further pertains to the downward movement of Body Fluids by the Lungs.

Impairment of the Lung's descending function will lead to Ki and body fluids becoming 'stuck' in the thorax, causing coughing and a congested feeling in the chest.

As we have seen, the Lungs play an important role in the distribution of Body Fluids. First, they disperse the Body Fluids throughout the periphery of the body, and secondly, they descend the Body Fluids to the Kidneys and Bladder. For this reason, they are considered to regulate the water passages. Failure of the Lungs to adequately disperse and descend Body Fluids often leads to slight water retention in the face.

Regulate the Water Passages

Because the Lungs disperse the Ki and ensure that the body surface receives adequate nourishment and moisture, the Lungs are said to control the skin and hair. If the Body Fluids are properly dispersed by the Lungs, the skin will be lustrous and the hair shiny. If not, the skin will become dry and body hair brittle and withered.

Control the Skin and Hair

The Lungs open into the nose, the gateway of the breath. When the Lungs are invaded by an external pathogenic factor, the nose easily becomes blocked and there is frequent sneezing. Sneezing is a sign that the descending of Lung-Ki is being obstructed.

Open into the Nose

Finally, the Lungs house the Corporeal Soul. We have already looked at the nature of the Corporeal Soul and the way in which it is affected by Grief. Feelings of sadness will also constrict the Corporeal Soul. This will in turn inhibit breathing and therefore blunt vitality. Otherwise, the Corporeal Soul is naturally optimistic and open to new experiences.

House the Corporeal Soul

THE FUNCTIONS OF THE LARGE INTESTINES

The functions of the Large Intestines are very simple: it receives food and drink from the Small Intestines, absorbs the remaining 'clean' fluids, and excretes the 'dirty' portion of food in the form of stools.

If the Lungs fail in their descending function, the Large Intestines may not receive sufficient Ki to ensure defecation. This will give rise to constipation, which is common with elderly people in whom Lung-Ki is often deficient.

Western naturopathic medicine recognizes that a loss of its appropriate bacterial colonization in the Large Intestines undermines health and weakens the immune system. Oriental Medicine also makes a connection between a healthy Large Intestine and the strength of the Defensive (Wei) Ki.

SHIATSU TREATMENT OF THE LUNGS

Weakness of Lung-Ki can develop as a result of spending long hours

Lung-Ki Deficiency

stooped over a desk. It can also come about through repeated chest infections which have not been properly treated, allowing External Wind to penetrate deeper into the Lungs.

Deficiency of Lung-Ki is apparent from a lack of vitality, shortness of breath, a weak voice, spontaneous sweating and possibly cough. The face will have a bright, white colour. Such a condition will also lead to a deficiency of Defensive Ki, resulting in the frequent occurrence of respiratory infections. The pulse will be Empty and the tongue pale.

Check for a Kyo condition of the Lung Channel, and possibly the Heart Channel as well. Administer tonifying Shiatsu treatment if the Kyo condition is confirmed, concentrating on the Tsubos Lung-9, Lung-7 and Bladder-13, all of which tonify Lung-Ki.

Lung-Yin Deficiency

When the Yin of the Lungs are deficient, one sees symptoms of Yin-deficiency (feelings of heat, a dry mouth and throat, thirst, insomnia, night sweats and so on) together with symptoms which indicate a Lung problem. These include a dry cough with very little mucus, sputum tinged with blood, and a hoarse voice. The pulse will be Floating; the tongue will be red, dry and possibly peeled or cracked in the Lung area.

It is again necessary to check whether the Lung Channel is Kyo in condition, together with that of the Kidneys, as the Kidneys are the source of Yin in the body. Shiatsu treatment should again be tonifying in nature, and include the Tsubos Lung-9, and Bladder-43, both of which tonify Lung-Yin. Kidney-Yin may be strengthened through the tonification of the Tsubo Kidney-6.

Invasion of the Lungs by Wind

The Lungs are considered to be the most exterior Organ of the body and have a strong influence on the Defensive Ki. When External pathogenic Wind invades the Defensive level of the body, the resulting struggle between the invading Wind and the Defensive Ki leads to fever. The Lungs' dispersing and descending function becomes impaired and causes the usual symptoms of a cold: cough, sneezing and blocked sinuses and so on. One feels tired and achy. Symptoms involving External Wind can be classified according to Cold and Hot types.

Wind-Cold is in evidence when the body feels chilled and mildly feverish, when nasal mucus is clear and watery, the throat is itchy, and there is an absence of thirst and sweating. Headaches arising from Wind-Cold are centred on the back of the head. The tongue is covered by a thin, white coating.

Wind-Heat is characterized by a stronger fever, nasal mucus which is yellow, and a sore, often swollen throat. There is usually thirst and sweating. Headaches arising from Wind-Heat are often more severe, and are not limited to the occiput. The tongue is covered by a thin, yellow coating.

Check for a Jitsu condition of the Lung, Large Intestine and Triple Heater Channels. These should be dispersed in order to release the

External Wind. Shiatsu Treatment should be concentrated around the upper back and chest area. The Tsubo Bladder-12 disperses External Wind of both the Cold and Hot type. Disperse Lung-7 in the case of Wind-Cold; Large Intestine-4 and Triple Heater-5 in the case of Wind-Heat. Dispersal of the Tsubo Gall Bladder-20 will relieve headaches due to the invasion of External Wind.

In the Creation Cycle of the Five Elements the Earth Element is mother to Metal. It is therefore common for excessive Dampness produced by the Spleen to collect in the Lungs. This tends to occur in people who eat a high proportion of Damp-forming foods such as dairy products, sugar and raw food.

Phlegm Obstructing the Lungs

The Phlegm that accumulates obstructs breathing and causes coughing and the expectoration of profuse amounts of whitish sputum. The chest feels congested, there is shortness of breath and the complexion is white and pasty. The pulse is Slippery and the tongue has a thick, white coating.

Phlegm which is retained in the Lungs for long periods of time tends to become Phlegm-Heat. This becomes apparent in the production of sputum which is thick and yellow or green. The resulting cough has a barking quality, and there is again shortness of breath.

Check the Lung and Spleen Channels for either a Jitsu or Kyo condition. Treat the Channels accordingly, concentrating on the chest, Kyo, despite the fact that the presence of Phlegm indicates a Full condition. Treat the Channels accordingly concentrating on the chest, upper back and upper Hara. Specific Tsubos should include Lung-5 (for expelling Phlegm and Heat from the Lungs), Lung-7 (stimulating Lung descending function and stopping cough), Stomach-40 (excellent for clearing Phlegm) and Bladder-13 and -20 (Lung and Spleen Yu Points).

Symptomatic relief of obstruction by Phlegm can also be achieved by Shiatsu applied directly to the rib cage (see p.112).

SHIATSU TREATMENT OF THE LARGE INTESTINES

Problems which are common to the Large Intestines, such as constipation and diarrhoea, frequently find their root in other Organs, particularly the Liver and Spleen. Like the Lungs, the Large Intestines can also be invaded by external pathogenic factors such as Heat and Cold.

This problem arises from eating too many greasy foods, allowing Dampness to build-up in the Large Intestines. Again, Dampness may turn to Damp-Heat over a certain period of time. The problem is characterized by diarrhoea, burning in the anus, strong-smelling stools,

Damp-Heat in the Large Intestines

abdominal pain, fever, thirst and a feeling of heaviness.

Check the Large Intestine, Spleen and Stomach Channels for either a Jitsu or Kyo condition. As the problem is Full in nature, they are more likely to be Jitsu in condition. Treat them accordingly, giving particular attention to treatment of the Hara. Specific Tsubos should include Stomach-25 (Bo Point of the Large Intestine; stops diarrhoea), Spleen-6 and -9 (clear Dampness from the Lower Heater) and Large Intestine-11 (clears Heat from the bowels).

Cold Invading the Large Intestines

This problem arises when the Large Intestines are invaded by External Cold. It occurs when a person has been exposed to cold weather without sufficient clothing to keep the Hara warm. Invasion of Cold is characterized by acute abdominal pain, diarrhoea and feelings of cold, especially in the abdomen.

Check the Large Intestine and Stomach Channel for a Jitsu condition, as the problem is Full in nature and will invariably require dispersal. Concentrate treatment on these Channels and on the Hara. Disperse the Tsubos Stomach-25 (Bo Point of the Large Intestines) and Stomach-36 (excellent for expelling Cold).

THE SPIRIT OF METAL

The Metal Element reflects both the capacity to be involved and responsive as well as that of being detached and separate. Its dual nature is like the breath: expanding and contracting, receiving and releasing. It teaches us to partake of life, but without trying to 'hold on to it'. It diminishes our sense of 'I' and, according to Ted Kaptchuk, teaches us the Virtue of Reverence.

Learning reverence and respect for the body are important aspects of healing. We so often seem to live to gratify our mind and senses, often at the expense of good health. Cultivating the body revitalizes mind and Spirit and fosters openness and optimism.

The essentials of competent Shiatsu which reflect the qualities of Metal are positive connection and steadiness of breath. Establishing a vital connection with the recipient allows for the maximum transmission of Ki, and enhances the feeling of communication inherent in Shiatsu. Steadiness of breath ensures an empty mind, both of which are prerequisites for a strong and open Hara.

Chapter 16

Kyo/Jitsu, Symptoms and Organ Function

Shizuto Masunaga presented a list of symptoms for the Kyo and Jitsu conditions of each major Channel. The symptoms he categorized were based on his own clinical observations and interpretation of Oriental Medicine and Western physiology. Although he firmly established Kyo/Jitsu methodology as a tool of diagnosis in its own right, the many different physical and psychological symptoms which he ascribed to it were not always clearly explained.

As a means of summarizing the functions and disharmonies of the Organs, we have taken many of the key physical and psychological symptoms listed by Masunaga, and explained them in a way that demonstrates their direct relationship to Organ function according to Oriental Medicine.

KYO/JITSU AND SYMPTOMS OF THE YIN ORGANS

Kidney Kyo

Symptom	*Explanation*
Chronic fatigue	Kidneys are the root of Yang
Excessive urination	Kidneys control Water
Poor circulation in the hips and Hara	Kidneys warm the Lower Heater
Lower back ache	Kidneys warm the Lower Heater; Kidney Marrow fills the spine
Weak sexual vitality	Kidney-Essence governs reproduction and harmonizes sexual function; Kidney-Yang mobilizes Essence
Brittle/soft bones	Kidney Marrow controls the bones

Symptoms	Explanation
Poor nails	Kidney Marrow helps make Blood
Thirst/dry mouth and throat	Kidney-Yin deficiency
Anxiety/restlessness/insomnia	Kidneys fail to anchor the Mind; Kidney-Yin deficiency
Lack of will/endurance	Kidneys fail to house the Will (*Zhi*)
Fear/apprehension	Fear is the emotion of the Water Element

Kidney Jitsu

Symptom	Explanation
Thirst/dark urine/blood in the urine	Kidney-Yin deficiency causing Heat in the Kidneys
Nosebleeds/fainting/heaviness in head/bitter taste in mouth	Kidney-Yin deficiency causing rising Excess Yang
Inflamed throat	Kidney-Yin deficiency and Kidney-Heat leading to Lung-Heat
Ringing in the ears	Kidneys open into the ears; Kidney-Yin deficiency causing rising Yang
Back stiffness	Kidneys control the Lower Heater
Excessive sexual drive	Kidney-Yin deficiency
Impatience/restlessness/work-aholic	Kidney disharmony causing hyperactive Will (*Zhi*)

Liver Kyo

Symptom	Explanation
Fatigue/dizziness/dull pale complexion	Liver fails to store the Blood, causing Blood deficiency
Cracked nails	Liver-Blood manifests in the nails
Infertility	Liver-Blood important to nourish the Uterus
Weak eyes/'floaters' in the eyes	Liver-Blood fails to nourish the eyes

Symptoms	*Explanation*
Weak joints/stiff muscles	Liver controls the tendons ('sinews')
Irritability/depression	Depressed Liver Ki affects the emotions
Lack of determination/inconsistent	'Liver [in health] is a resolute Organ'

Liver Jitsu

Symptom	*Explanation*
Exhaustion due to excessive drive	'Liver is a resolute Organ'
Swollen epigastrium/poor digestion/flatulence	Liver Ki stagnation invades the Stomach
Headaches	Liver Ki stagnation/Liver-Yang rising
Chronic stiffness/tightness in Hara	Liver Ki stagnation affecting the sinews and muscles
Haemorrhoids/skin eruptions	Liver Heat transmitted to Blood
Inflammatory diseases of reproductive system	Liver Channel encircles genitals; Liver Fire
Excessive work and concentration/stubborn	'Liver is a resolute organ'
Frustrated/impatient/impulsive	Liver-Ki stagnation; Ki does not flow freely
Represses anger/explodes	Stagnation of the emotions

Heart Kyo

Symptom	*Explanation*
Poor circulation/fatigue	Heart governs Blood and circulation
Palpitations/angina pectoris	Deficiency of Heart-Yang, -Yin or -Blood
Stuttering/pulling sensation in the tongue	Heart opens into the tongue
Sweaty palms	Heart controls sweat
Weakness/tightness in upper Hara	Upper Hara is Heart diagnostic area
Nervous tension/over-sensitivity/shock	Heart houses the Mind (Shen)

Symptoms	*Explanation*
Anxiety/restlessness	Heart-Yin deficiency
Poor memory	Heart-Blood deficiency
Sadness/disappointment	Joy is the emotion of the Fire Element

Heart Jitsu

Symptom	*Explanation*
Palpitations/chest pain	Heart-Blood stagnation/Heart-Fire blazing
Poor circulation	Heart-Blood stagnation
Ulcers on the tongue	Heart opens into the tongue; Heart-Fire blazing
Heavy perspiration	Heart controls sweat
Stiffness/fullness in the upper Hara	Heart diagnostic area
Nervousness/restlessness/over-excitement	Heart houses the Mind (Shen); excessive 'Joy'
Hysteria/mania/excessive, inappropriate laughter	Full condition of the Heart; a Mind agitated by Heat or Fire

Heart Governor Kyo

Symptoms	*Explanation*
Palpitations/breathless on exertion/weak pulse	Deficient Ki of the Heart and Heart Governor
Poor circulation and cold limbs	Deficient Yang of Heart and Heart Governor
Anxiety/restlessness/insomnia	Deficient Yin of Heart and Heart Governor
Emotional over-sensitivity in relationships	Heart Governor influences close relating

Heart Governor Jitsu

Symptoms	*Explanation*
Constriction, stuffiness and heaviness in the chest	Blood stagnation of Heart and Heart Governor
Palpitations/tongue and mouth ulcers/insomnia/heat	Fire in the Heart and Heart Governor

Symptoms	Explanation
Over-emotional/impulsive/ agitated, particularly in regard to relationships	Excessive 'Joy' and excitement

Spleen Kyo

Symptom	Explanation
Poor digestion/emaciation/ appetite loss/lethargy	Spleen's transformation function impaired
Accumulation of catarrh and phlegm	Spleen's transformation function impaired
Heavy, tired limbs	Spleen controls the muscles and four limbs
Anaemia	Spleen is the origin of Blood
Lack of saliva/lack of taste	Spleen opens into the mouth/fails to raise fluids
Pale gums	Spleen opens into the mouth
Prolapse	Spleen's raising of Ki function fails
Sleepiness	Spleen fails to raise Ki/Spleen Dampness affects head
Overthinking/worry/poor concentration	Spleen is the residence of Thought (Yi)
Craves sympathy and understanding	Spleen requires nurturing/is the Organ of consideration

Spleen Jitsu

Symptom	Explanation
Appetite loss/gastric hyperacidity	Spleen's transformation function impaired: accumulation of Phlegm-Heat
Sticky feeling in mouth/mucus in the Lungs	Poor transformation leads to Phlegm-Damp
Obesity	Poor transformation leads to Dampness and oedema
Heaviness in the legs/stiffness in the arms/lack of strength	Spleen controls the muscles and four limbs
Overthinking/obsessiveness/un- clear thinking	Spleen is the residence of Thought (Yi)

Symptoms	Explanation
Excessive concern for others/self-pity	Spleen is the Organ of nurturing/excessive Thought becomes worry

Lung Kyo

Symptom	Explanation
Difficulty breathing/cough/bronchitis	Lungs govern respiration
Fatigue, especially in upper body	Lungs govern Ki
Frequent colds/influenza	Lungs govern dispersing and descending function/Defensive Ki
Heaviness in the head	Lungs control the Channels and blood vessels
Unenthusiastic, negative attitude	Lungs house Corporeal Soul ($P'o$) source of one's vital spirit
Grief/melancholy	Grief is the emotion of the Metal Element

Lung Jitsu

Symptom	Explanation
Nasal and chest congestion	Phlegm-Damp obstructing the Lungs
Coughing pain in the chest	Full condition of the Lungs
Bronchitis	Heat and Phlegm in the Lungs
Asthma	Impairment of the Lungs dispersing and descending function
Tight chest/muscles	Stagnation of Ki in the chest
Pulling sensation in thumb	Lung Channel obstruction
Grief/oppression	Grief is the emotion of the Metal Element
Detachment/defensiveness/pride	Inability to 'open up'
Selfishness/jealousy	Inability to 'let go'

KYO/JITSU AND SYMPTOMS OF THE YANG ORGANS

Bladder Kyo

Symptom	*Explanation*
Frequent, pale, copious urination	Bladder fails to properly transform fluids due to Kidney-Yang deficiency
Incontinence	Bladder fails to control fluids due to Kidney-Yang deficiency
Poor circulation in the Hara and legs/cold and achy lower back	Kidney Yang fails to warm Lower Heater/Bladder deficiency with Cold
Fear and apprehension	Fear is the emotion of the Water Element

Bladder Jitsu

Symptom	*Explanation*
Frequent, urgent urination/difficult urination	Dampness in the Bladder obstructs the flow of fluids
Turbid, milky urine	Dampness in the Bladder
Heaviness and cramping in lower Hara	Dampness and Cold in the Bladder
Burning urination/blood in the urine	Heat in the Bladder
Tightness in the back of the legs	Obstruction of Bladder Channel
Jealousy and suspicion	Fear/inability to 'let go'

Gall Bladder Kyo

Symptom	*Explanation*
Dizziness/poor vision	Part of Liver-Blood deficiency pattern
Poor digestion of fats	Impairment of Gall Bladder function of bile secretion
Weak, tired legs	Gall Bladder Channel has an important influence on the legs
Timidity and lack of initiative	Gall Bladder is the source of courage

Gall Bladder Jitsu

Symptom	*Explanation*
Pain and swelling under rib cage/nausea/loss of appetite	Dampness in the Gall Bladder/ Stagnation of Liver-Ki
Poor digestion of fats/yellow complexion	Secretion of bile obstructed by Dampness
Bitter taste in the mouth/dark urine	Heat/inflammation in the Gall Bladder
Gallstones	'Substantial' Phlegm obstructs the Gall Bladder
Stiff muscles along sides of body	Obstruction of Gall Bladder Channel
Impatient/hurried/driven/over-ambitious	Initiative and 'courage' in excess
Irritable/frustrated/angry	Anger is the emotion of the Wood Element

Small Intestines Kyo

Symptom	*Explanation*
Abdominal pain/desire for hot drinks	Cold in the Small Intestines obstructs Ki-flow in abdomen – caused by Spleen-Yang Deficiency
Borborygmi (gurgling in the abdomen)	Characteristic of Small Intestines disharmony
Diarrhoea	Small Intestines and Spleen fail to transform food and drink due to Yang Deficiency
Lack of strength in Hara/poor circulation in hips	Deficiency of Small Intestines; poor Ki-flow in Lower Heater
Shoulder pain	Obstruction of Small Intestines Channel
Indecision/lack of mental clarity	Small Intestines separates the pure from the impure

Small Intestines Jitsu

Symptoms	*Explanation*
Abdominal swelling/twisting pain in abdomen	Stagnation of Ki in the Small Intestines, caused by Liver-Ki stagnation

Symptoms	*Explanation*
Borborygmi/flatulence/constipation	Ki Stagnation impairs transformation function of Small Intestines
Abdominal pain with signs of Heat/thirst/restlessness/dark, scanty urine	Heat in the Small Intestines
Deafness	Fire in the Small Intestine Channel
Stiffness and pain in the shoulders and neck	Obstruction of the Small Intestine Channel
Mental restlessness/obsessiveness/indecision	Small Intestine separates the pure from the impure/influences the Heart and hence the Mind

Triple Heater Kyo

Symptoms	*Explanation*
Feelings of cold	Triple Heater fails to distribute warmth from the Gate of Vitality
Susceptibility to colds and flu	Ki deficiency of the Upper Heater
Abdominal swelling/indigestion/loose stools	Impairment of function of the Middle Heater
Oedema, swelling and Cold in the lower abdomen	Impairment of function of the Lower Heater
Socially unconfident/recluse	Exterior relationship to Heart Governor, influencing social communication
Unadventurous/timid	Lack of 'Joy'

Triple Heater Jitsu

Symptoms	*Explanation*
Earache/lateral headache/swollen cheeks/sore throat	External Wind invades the Triple Heater Channel
Indigestion/abdominal pain and heaviness	Stagnant Ki and Retention of Food in the Middle Heater
Constipation/fullness and tightness in the Hara	Stagnant Ki in the Lower Heater

Symptoms	*Explanation*
Tightness and tension in the arms, shoulders and neck	Obstruction of the Triple Heater Channel
Socially tense/over-cautious	Triple Heater influences wider social relationships and when in harmony reflects extroverted aspects of Fire Element

Stomach Kyo

Symptoms	*Explanation*
Stomach discomfort/lack of appetite and taste/tired in the morning	Stomach-Ki deficiency
Vomiting of clear fluid/cold limbs/loose stools	Stomach-Ki deficiency with Cold
Lack of appetite/dull epigastric pain/fullness after eating/Heat signs	Stomach-Yin deficiency
Overthinking/worry/poor concentration	Pensiveness is the 'emotion' of the Earth Element
Despondent/apathetic	No 'appetite' for life

Stomach Jitsu

Symptoms	*Explanation*
Fullness and swelling in the Stomach/bad breath/lack of appetite	Retention of Food in the Stomach due to stagnant Ki
Belching/'heartburn'/hiccups/vomiting	Stomach Ki rebelling upwards due to stagnant Ki
Burning pain in the Stomach/thirst for cold drinks/hunger/bleeding gums	Fire and Phlegm in the Stomach
Stiffness on the anterior surfaces of the leg	Obstruction of Stomach Channel
Over-thinking/obsessiveness	Pensiveness is the 'emotion' of the Earth Element
Mania/manic depression	Excessive Stomach Heat and Phlegm agitates and clouds the Mind

Large Intestines Kyo

Symptoms	*Explanation*
Loose stools/borborygmi/dull pain in the abdomen/cold limbs	Cold in the Large Intestines, associated with Spleen-Yang deficiency
Haemorrhoids	Spleen-Yang deficiency leads to collapse of Large Intestines
Dry stools/constipation	Lack of fluids in Large Intestines due to general Yin/Blood deficiency
Lack of strength in the thumb	Obstruction of Large Intestines Channel
Disappointment/melancholy	Grief is the emotion of the Metal Element
Unenthusiastic/pessimistic/no 'spirit'	Large Intestines related, through the Lungs, to the Corporeal Soul, source of vitality

Large Intestines Jitsu

Symptoms	*Explanation*
Diarrhoea/mucus in stools/burning anus/abdominal pain	Damp-Heat in the Large Intestines
Constipation with dry stools/burning anus/dry, burning mouth	Heat in the Large Intestines
Swelling in the lower Hara	Dampness in the Large Intestines
Remorse/depression	Grief is the emotion of the Metal Element
Worry which cannot be released	Inability to 'let go'

PART 3

SHIATSU DIAGNOSIS

This section deals with systematic methods for assessing levels of health and disharmony. This enables us to build up a picture of the recipient's constitution and condition, so that we can deduce the underlying cause of their disharmony and decide upon the optimum mode of treatment.

The *Nan Ching* (Chapter 61, p.43) suggests a general approach including some or all of the following procedures:

1. Look at and watch the patient.
2. Listen to and smell the patient.
3. Ask the patient questions.
4. Touch the patient.

Chapter 17

Looking Diagnosis

Immediately the client comes into sight we can get an overall impression of them. We can discern their constitutional body type; see whether or not there is a general Fullness or Emptiness in the upper or lower half of their body; make deductions from colour hues on the face, facial markings, blemishes and other visible features. With experience, these can be discerned at a glance.

CONSTITUTIONAL BODY TYPES

Generally an 'excess' body will tend to have tight musculature, compared to a 'deficient' type body which will have soft flesh and poor circulation.

The following presents archetypes within the Five Elements, although we must realize that pure archetypes are rare, and most people are made up of a combination of several Element types.

Water – Soft features. Often dark or bluish complexion. Tends to be lazy, slow and adaptable.

Wood – Hard, tight and strong musculature. Greenish or purplish complexion. Organized, possibly tense. Sudden rigid movement.

Fire – Fine pointed features. Wide forehead and high cheekbones. Red complexion. Sometimes nervous. Adventurous.

Earth – Heavy set, often flaccid. Tendency to be overweight. Sallow, yellow complexion. Slow moving, calm and practical.

Metal – Broad shouldered, but often hollow-chested and lean. White, pale complexion. Careful in movement, enjoying stillness. Rational and slightly melancholic.

POLARITY OF FULL OR EMPTY

A person may present an overall picture of Fullness manifesting as predominant *Jitsu* in the body, or they may present a sense of Emptiness by appearing predominantly *Kyo*. With a predominantly Jitsu or Kyo person it is sometimes possible to see a discrepancy between the upper and lower half of the body. This requires a trained eye, but is something which comes very quickly with practice. Obviously it is clearer if the discrepancy is extreme. Below are some exaggerated possibilities plus broad principles for re-establishing harmony (based on author's clinical observations).

A. Predominantly *Jitsu* with upper body more Jitsu than lower body

General approach: dispersal techniques over entire body, concentrating more on upper half. Find most Kyo area/Channel in lower body and tonify (reaction is often rapid).

B. Predominantly *Jitsu* with lower body more Jitsu than upper body

General approach: dispersal techniques over entire body, concentrating more on lower half. Find most Kyo area/Channel in upper body and tonify (reaction is often rapid, though slower than A).

Fig. 17.1: Right
Predominantly Jitsu, upper body more Jitsu than lower

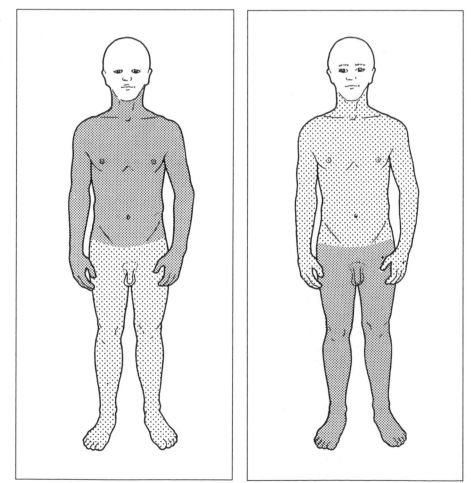

Fig. 17.2: Far right
Predominantly Jitsu, lower body more Jitsu than upper

General approach: find most Kyo area/Channel in upper body and tonify (reaction is often considerably slower than Jitsu condition).

C. Predominantly *Kyo* with upper body more Kyo than lower body

General approach: find most Kyo area/Channel in lower body and tonify. This condition generally indicates the weakest condition of the Hara. Therefore holding and tonifying the Hara is effective (reaction usually slow).

D. Predominantly *Kyo* with lower body more Kyo than upper body

Remember that generally, Kyo should be tonified before Jitsu is dispersed. However, sometimes it is necessary to first disperse some Jitsu to reveal the underlying Kyo. This often applies in examples A and B above.

Occasionally you see a major discrepancy between front and back, so that the anterior of the trunk is very Kyo, while the back is Jitsu, or vice versa. Front Jitsu/back Kyo relates to a person who desperately wants to appear strong and able to cope, but whose actual energy reserves are

Fig. 17.3: Far left Predominantly Kyo, upper body more Kyo than lower

Fig. 17.4: Left Predominantly Kyo, lower body more Kyo than upper very limited. These people need tonification on their back and extensive work on their hara. Back Jitsu/front Kyo can indicate a timid, nervous person. Tonification of the Kidney Channel in the chest, plus general tonification of the Hara is very beneficial. Bear in mind that it may require patience to have the receiver feel secure enough to open their Hara to you.

Left/right discrepancies are much more likely when structural imbalances, previous injury or dis-eased organ pathology are present. First check whether the structural imbalance is a skeletal discrepancy, such as a shorter bone on one side of the body, or energetic. If it is not a fixed skeletal problem then tonification of the Kyo channels on the Kyo side is required. The Gall Bladder Channel is often involved.

THE FACE

Complexion Because the Stomach is the source of body fluids, a complexion which is dull or dry looking indicates depleted Stomach Ki, whereas strong Ki is reflected in a clear and moist complexion.

Colour
White – General deficiency and Cold
Red – Heat
Yellow – Spleen deficiency and/or Dampness
Green – Liver disharmony, internal cold or pain
Black Blue – Cold, pain or Kidney disease

Face Areas There are numerous sources of literature exhibiting considerable differences in the correspondences associated with areas on the face. Fig. 17.5 illustrates those areas of facial correspondences born out by our clinical experience.

FACIAL DIAGNOSTIC AREAS

Kidneys Located in the area directly beneath the eyes. Dark rings under the eyes generally indicate weakness of Kidney function. Puffiness indicates Kidney-Yang deficiency. Sunken red hollows may indicate Kidney-Yin deficiency. The condition of the Kidneys may also be revealed through their close link with the ears; redness of the ears often indicates the presence of Heat in the Kidneys.

Liver Located between the eyebrows. Furrows between the eyebrows indicate long-term Liver Ki stagnation. A red patch here indicates Liver-Heat or

Liver-Fire.

Corresponds to the eyelids. Redness of the eyelids may indicate Heat in **Gall Bladder**
the Gall Bladder.

Located on the tip of the nose. A swollen tip indicates a weak Heart **Heart**
function. A red swollen tip may indicate Heat in the Heart.

Located on the inside corner of the eye socket, on the temples and on the **Spleen**
upper bridge of the nose. Darkness and discoloration on the inside
corner of the eye socket indicates Spleen weakness. Yellow discoloration
on the upper bridge of the nose and temples indicates weakness in the
Spleen's transformative function. A vertical line crossing the upper
bridge of the nose between the eyes also indicates long-standing Spleen
disharmony.

Located midway along the bridge of the nose and on the upper lip. A **Stomach**
yellow discoloration indicates weakness in the Stomach's digestive
function. A slight swelling of the upper lip may also indicate a Stomach
disharmony. Dryness and cracking of the upper lip may indicate
Stomach-Yin deficiency.

Located on the cheeks. A white discoloration indicates Lung-Ki and or **Lungs**
-Yang deficiency; a red discoloration may indicate Lung-Yin deficiency
or -Heat.

Corresponds to the nostrils. Redness of the nostrils indicates Heat in the **Bronchi**
bronchii.

Corresponds to the lower lip and the area around the base of the jaw. **Large Intestines**
Red skin eruptions in this area may indicate Damp-Heat in the Large
Intestines. Swelling of the lower lip may indicate weakness in the Large
Intestines' eliminative function, and therefore constipation. Dryness
may indicate a lack of body fluids in the intestines.

Located in the area around the mouth, between the nose and the chin. In **Reproductive Organs**
women, a purple discoloration in this area may indicate stagnation of Ki
in the Lower Heater, causing pre-menstrual tension and menstrual pain.
Red skin eruption in this area indicates Damp-Heat in the reproductive
organs.

Nervous System Located on the forehead. Bearing in mind the person's age, a large number of vertical lines may indicate weakness in the function of the nervous system.

Please note that these associations are very generalized and should be considered only in the light of a more general diagnosis, taking into account information provided by the patient's symptoms and tongue. For example, while red cheeks may indicate Heat in the Lungs, it may equally indicate overall Yin deficiency. Although we have linked the lips to the Stomach and Large Intestines, they may also reflect the condition of the Spleen as the 'Spleen opens onto the lips'. Despite the fact that the 'Kidneys open into the ears', the ears can also show the condition of the entire body.

Eyes The eyes reflect the state of the mind (Shen) and Essence (Jing). If the state of Mind and Essence is strong, the eyes will be clear and bright. If the Mind is disturbed and the Essence is weak, the eyes will be lustreless and cloudy.

Fig. 17.5: The face

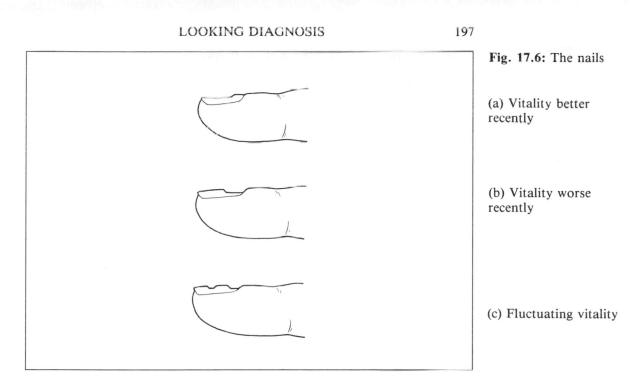

Fig. 17.6: The nails

(a) Vitality better recently

(b) Vitality worse recently

(c) Fluctuating vitality

NAILS

Moist and healthy nails reflect the vitality of the Liver. If there is deficient Liver-Blood to nourish the nails, they will become dry, dark, indented and possibly cracked. Concave nails reflect a chronic Lung Kyo condition.

A sudden decrease in Liver-Blood will result in a sudden decrease in nail thickness, allowing us to establish when the deficiency occurred, provided it was within the previous twelve months (fingernails take six months to grow; toenails take approximately twelve months). Conversely, restoration of nail thickness will tell us that Liver-Blood has been restored.

TOES AND FINGERS

Longstanding Kyo or Jitsu distortion in the Channels can often be seen to produce lateral or medial deviation of the toe into which the Channel flows. The fingers tend not to have these deviations because they are not confined and restricted like the toes.

A lateral deviation indicates Jitsu whereas medial deviation indicates Kyo. Jitsu can also cause a toe to cross over another toe, whereas Kyo can result in a toe dropping and crossing *under* another toe.

Spleen Kyo and Liver Jitsu could cause lateral deviation of the big toe, especially if there is chronic Spleen Kyo *and* Liver Jitsu. Medial deviation of the big toe and lateral deviation of the fifth toe is unlikely, due to the pressure of shoes against them.

A weak looking toe or finger with a narrow 'waist' indicates constitutional weakness in the Channels flowing into it.

Very chronic constipation commonly results in stiffness of the index fingers.

Fig. 17.7: Toes and fingers

(a) Lateral deviation of toe indicating chronic Stomach Jitsu

(b) Medial deviation of toe indicating chronic Gall Bladder Kyo

Fig. 17.8: Finger with narrow 'waist'

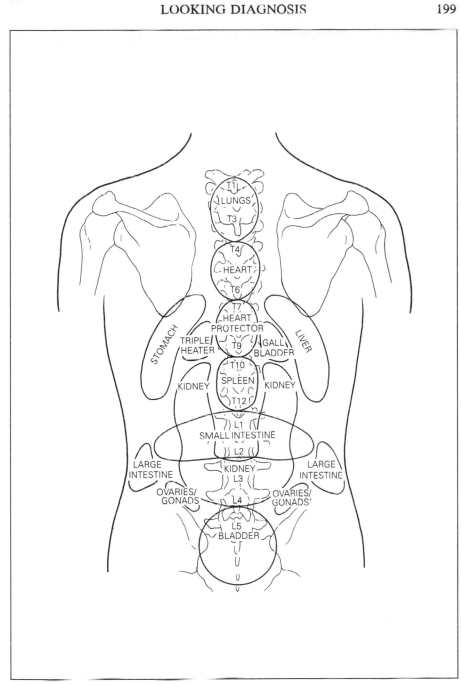

Fig. 17.9: Back Organ Correspondences by area

BACK DIAGNOSIS

With the recipient lying prone, relative Jitsu and Kyo areas can be seen. Do not adjust the receiver's clothing because folds and creases often highlight areas of imbalance. Jitsu will be seen to stand out whereas Kyo will seem flatter or more depressed than normal. With practice, marked skeletal imbalances such as excessive thoracic roundness (or kyphosis) cease to be a distraction. You might for example mistake thoracic kyphosis as Heart Protector Jitsu. As with touch, try to discern Kyo/Jitsu by the absence or presence of vitality.

Figure 17.9 shows the back area correspondences.

Kyo/Jitsu can also be seen along the Channels. For example, Bladder Jitsu is really noticeable where it runs either side of the spinal column, in the buttock and along the back of the legs.

It is easier if the receiver wears plain-coloured clothing to avoid distractions. If you cannot see any obvious Kyo/Jitsu, covering the receiver with a white sheet will often highlight it. (Do explain to them first, or they may think the procedure rather strange.)

Chapter 18

Touch Diagnosis

Touch Diagnosis is the most important ingredient in the Shiatsu health assessment because the entire technique and purpose of Shiatsu is to touch. Therefore it is only natural that touch should be the primary diagnostic tool.

CHANNEL DIAGNOSIS

Excess or deficient Ki within the Channels can be felt as a Jitsu or Kyo quality as we apply Shiatsu technique to the Channels. The qualities of both Jitsu and Kyo have been discussed already on pp.17–19. In short, if the receiver feels your touch as dull sensation, dull soreness or ache, this indicates a Kyo condition. Sharp sensation such as sharp pain indicates a Jitsu condition. Each Channel will exhibit some areas of Jitsu and some of Kyo, although one will predominate. A total rebalance of Ki within the Channels could be achieved by working each Channel along its entire surface pathway, tonifying or dispersing Kyo and Jitsu wherever it is located. However, this would be a long, laborious process. Alternatively, each Channel could be stretched in the arms and legs using the techniques detailed in Chapter 6.

A Jitsu condition will feel hard, but with an elastic feel of resistance, whereas a Kyo condition will feel flabby, weak and often stiff if deeply penetrated. For maximum effectiveness, treatment can be administered to the most Kyo and the most Jitsu Channels.

HARA DIAGNOSIS

There are several facets to Hara diagnosis useful to Shiatsu practitioners.

This method enables us to find the most Kyo and most Jitsu Channels more quickly than direct palpation or stretching of the Channels. Figure **Zen Shiatsu Hara Diagnosis**

Fig. 18.1: Zen Shiatsu Hara diagnosis areas

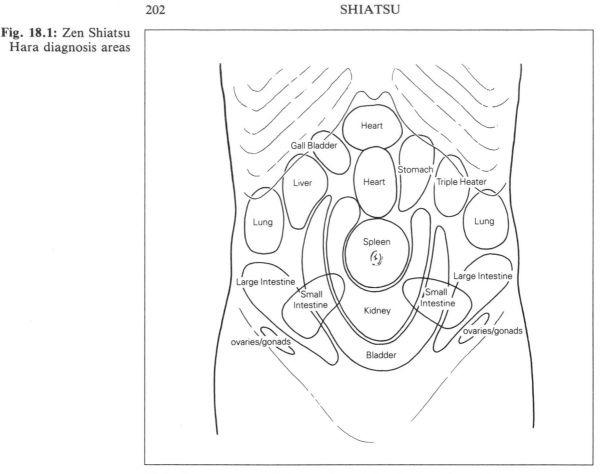

18.1 gives a map of the twelve abdominal areas which relate to the twelve major Channels. Kyo or Jitsu found in these areas will reflect the energetic state of the corresponding Channels.

There are three methods of applying this system, namely:

- Deep Touch Method
- Light Touch Method
- No Touch Method

The *deep touch method* requires moderately deep pressure for the purpose of locating pain, discomfort, tension, strength or weakness of the abdominal muscles, pulsing of blood vessels or lumps. Any of these observations can indicate by inference the interplay of Kyo/Jitsu. A sense of *reaction* indicates Jitsu, whereas *lack of reaction* signifies Kyo. Be careful to discount matter or gas in the intestines. If you feel any other lumps, especially if they feel like 'cauliflower', gently suggest that the client has it medically examined, if they have not already done so.

The *light touch method* is quicker and free from distractions by the abdominal contents. The diagnostic areas are scanned with the lightest

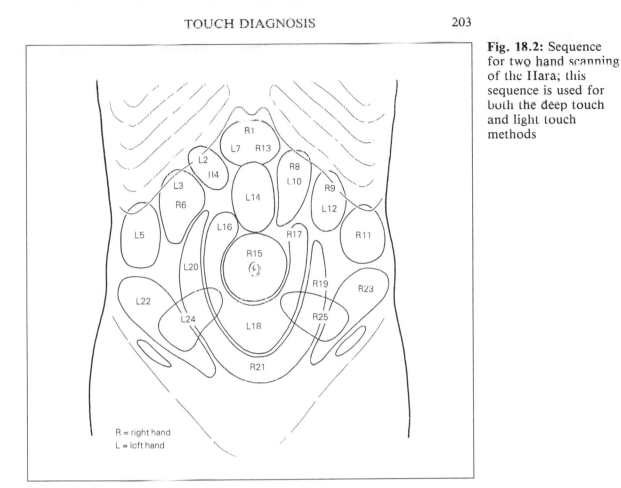

Fig. 18.2: Sequence for two hand scanning of the Hara; this sequence is used for both the deep touch and light touch methods

R = right hand
L = left hand

touch using the fingertips of both hands, in the sequence illustrated in Figure 18.2. This sequence enables each area to be contacted twice, thus allowing a constant comparison with an adjacent area or with the Heart area.

Once the most Kyo and most Jitsu areas have been discovered they can be checked by first holding the *Jitsu* area, then holding the *Kyo* area with the other hand. If the assessment is correct, there will be a definite feeling of connection and reaction between the two areas. In particular, the Jitsu area will feel like it is 'opening' or 'sinking'. If you get no reaction, try holding another Kyo area. Because the Jitsu area is easier to find, it is less likely to have been incorrectly diagnosed. Continue in this manner until you get a definite reaction.

This is a very subtle and consequently a very subjective approach, which works better if you trust your first impression. The longer you think about it and the more you try to cross check it, the more your analytical faculties will interfere with your sensitivity. This method is very 'Zen', in that the less you struggle for an answer, the more likely the answer will come.

Making a quick decision is also necessary in this instance, because the more you pad around on the Hara, the more likely you are to initiate an energetic change, and therefore arrive at a reading which is modified by your touch.

The *no touch method* involves passing your palms over each area at a distance of 2–4 inches. For this method, you need to be sensitive to the etheric field of Ki around the body, which although sounding esoteric, is in fact easier and more tangible for many people than discerning Kyo/Jitsu through touch. As you move your hand slowly you can feel sensations of heat, cold, or what feels like an updraught of wind. Heat and/or an updraught of wind indicate Jitsu. Cold often indicates Kyo. A feeling of uniformity, like riding on a carpet of air, is a sign of natural health. Feelings of an empty hole in this 'carpet' indicate Kyo. This method, when mastered, enables you quickly to narrow down the entire energetic distortions to the deepest underlying Kyo deficiency.

It is common for the Kyo/Jitsu reading to be different on the Hara compared to the reading on the Back. This does not mean that each method is in contradiction to the other, but that they each illustrate different depths of the receiver's energetic imbalances. The Back is usually considered to display more chronic imbalances whereas the Hara indicates more acute imbalances. With experience, however, the Hara reading can indicate the deepest underlying imbalance. Whether you treat according to the Hara or the Back will depend on which level of the recipient's problem you wish to tackle on that particular occasion, and to some extent on which of your senses you believe to be the most reliable and clear; the visual or the tactile.

Five Reflex Hara Diagnosis

This system is less precise, but can be used to indicate broadly marked imbalances in any of the Five Elements. Indications in this system tend to manifest on a much more physical level in the form of 'abdominal masses'. Abdominal masses that move under fingertip pressure indicate stagnation of Ki. Hard masses that do not move indicate stasis of Blood.

Note that all the correspondences along the vertical midline are similar to the Zen Shiatsu system (see Fig. 18.3).

Other Indications from the Hara

- The upper Hara just below the xiphoid process and Directing Vessel-15 should be looser than the rest. If if feels hard and knotted it indicates a constraint of Heart and Lung Ki. The lower Hara below the umbilicus and around Directing Vessel-6 should feel elastic but firmer and tighter than the rest. If it feels soft and flabby it indicates a weakness of the Original Ki which resides between the Kidneys to activate all physiological functions and to provide heat for digestion. To strengthen the lower Hara and Original Ki, tonification should be applied to the Kidney and Triple Heater channels. (The Triple Heater is the 'avenue' for the Original Ki, distributing it to all the organs and ultimately to all the channels.)

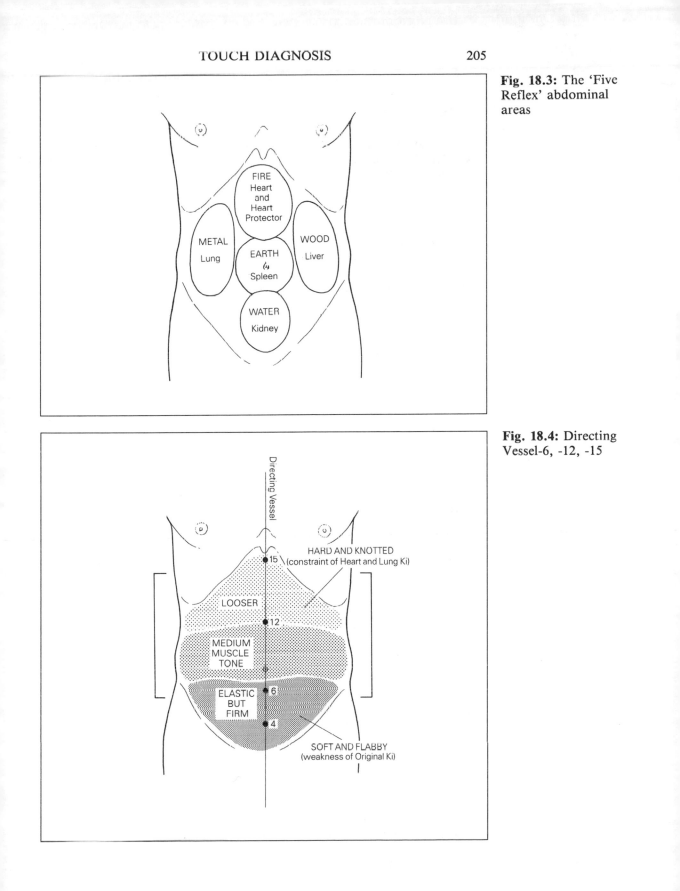

Fig. 18.3: The 'Five Reflex' abdominal areas

FIRE
Heart
and
Heart
Protector

METAL
Lung

EARTH
&
Spleen

WOOD
Liver

WATER
Kidney

Fig. 18.4: Directing Vessel-6, -12, -15

Directing Vessel

HARD AND KNOTTED
(constraint of Heart and Lung Ki)

15

LOOSER

12

MEDIUM
MUSCLE
TONE

ELASTIC
BUT
FIRM

6

4

SOFT AND FLABBY
(weakness of Original Ki)

The mid Hara above the umbilicus, around Directing Vessel-12, should have less tightness than Directing Vessel-6, but be firmer than Directing Vessel-15 (see Fig. 18.4).

- A painful Hara is a sign of deficient Spleen and Kidneys.
- The Directing Vessel line should be slightly depressed and lower than the Kidney and Stomach Channel lines (like a shallow valley). If it is raised above the Kidney and Stomach line, and especially distended around Directing Vessel-12, a weak Hara is indicated.
- Tension or spasm in the abdominal muscles when the Hara is in a relaxed position signifies deficient Kidney (and sometimes Spleen) Ki.
- An umbilicus which is close to the surface indicates a weaker Hara than if the umbilicus is deeply set. Strong pulsing around the umbilicus indicates deficient Spleen Ki. If the pulse is not central within the umbilicus, postural irregularities may be present. For example, if the pulse is to the left of the umbilicus, check for tightness and constriction on the left side of the torso.
- If there is pulsing below the sternum, which reaches down to the umbilicus, Heart and Kidney deficiency is indicated.

THE BACK TRANSPORTING POINTS

The Back Transporting Points are also known as Yu Points (Japanese) or Shu Points (Chinese). They are useful in diagnosis because they become tender on pressure when their associated Organ is ailing.

They are also very useful in the treatment of chronic disease. In addition they can be used to treat the sense organs of the corresponding visceral organs. The specific action of each Back Transporting Point is given under the discussion of Tsubos on p.237. Fig. 18.5 gives the location and associated Organ of these points.

THE FRONT COLLECTING POINTS

The Front Collecting Points are also known as Bo Points (Japanese) or Mu Points (Chinese). Like the Back Transporting Points, these points become tender when their associated Organ is ailing.

In treatment they have a regulating effect upon the internal Organs. They are useful in both acute and chronic dysfunction although they are more often used in acute cases.

Figure 18.6 gives the location and associated organ of these Points.

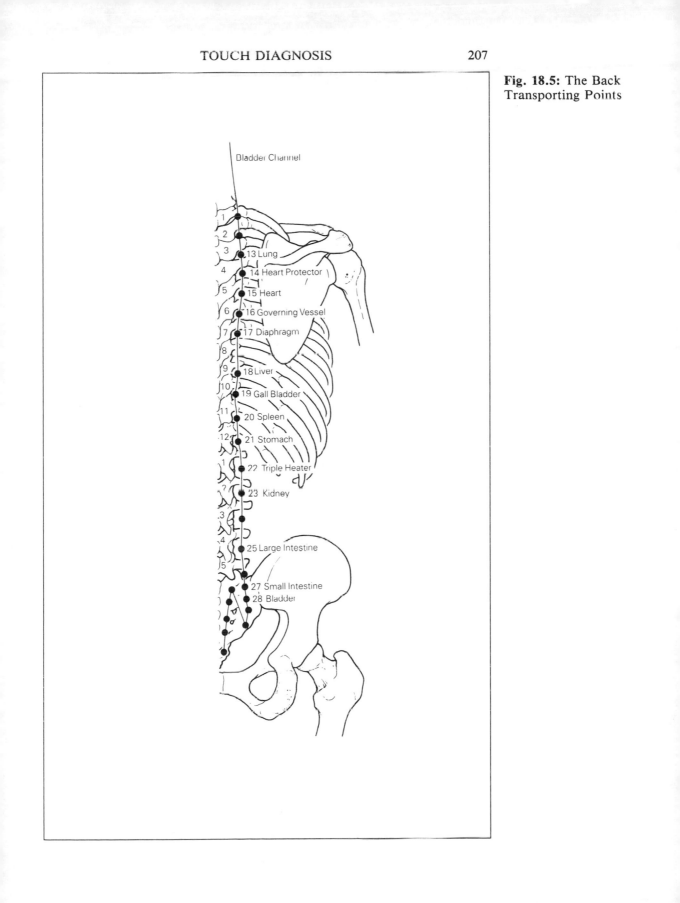

Fig. 18.6: The Front Collecting Points

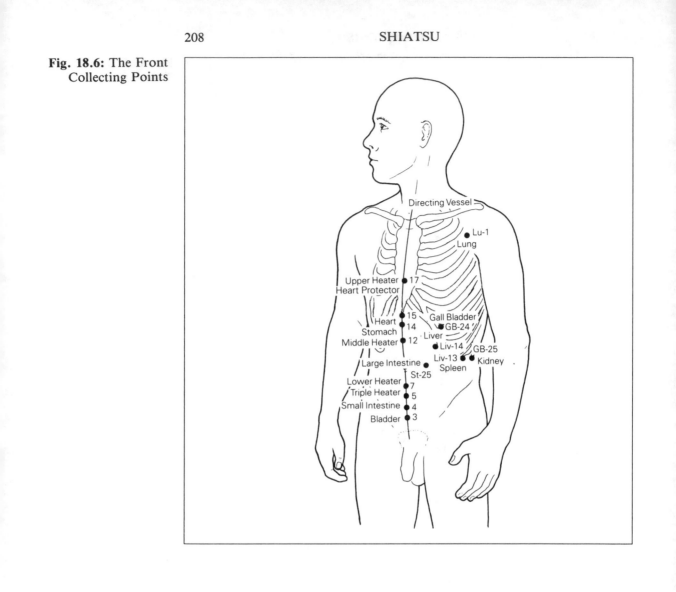

Chapter 19

Diagnosis Through Listening and Smelling

The relatively subtle diagnostic techniques of listening and smelling provide us with information gleaned from the sound of a client's voice and breathing, and the natural odour of their body.

The voice can be a fascinating source of insight into the emotional disposition of an individual. Like the emotions, the different sounds of the voice are categorized according to the Five Elements, and therefore offer information about the client's constitutional make-up. This means that the condition of Elements and Organs to which they point reveals potential, not necessarily actual, energetic problems. The sound of the voice should not generally be relied upon to provide us with information regarding the client's current physical condition.

The Sound of the Voice

When attempting to discern the underlying sound of the voice, one must focus one's attention away from both the subject matter being spoken of as well as the style or accent of the voice. This may take practice: one can first listen to the voices of fellow students and friends with the eyes closed, as they read aloud subject matter which will not distract.

The Kidneys give depth to the voice. However, the Water Element in disharmony will produce a groaning sound, especially discernible at the end of words and phrases. It may reveal a tendency towards feeling threatened or insecure.

The Liver gives the voice a sense of authority. When the Wood Element is affected there will be the presence of a shout in the voice. Alternatively, the person's voice may possess a clipped quality. A propensity towards feeling frustrated and angry is naturally indicated.

Ruling the tongue, the Heart ensures that words are well articulated. Speech impediments such as stuttering often reflect an energetic imbalance of the Heart. The Heart also gives a sense of buoyancy to the voice. When there is a tremulous quality to the voice, traditionally described as a Laugh, a problem with the Fire Element may be indicated. The person is likely to be prone to over-excitement or anxiety.

The Spleen gives a singing quality to the voice. A voice that has a singing sound which overrides all other qualities means that a disharmony of the Earth Element is probable. The person may tend to worry a lot.

Finally, the Lungs give strength to the voice. A voice which is weak may indicate Lung deficiency. Moreover, an underlying weeping sound in the voice may point to a problem with the Metal Element, and reveal a corresponding presence of sadness or Grief.

Finally, it must be stressed that, just as an individual possesses a number of predominating emotions, a voice may contain more than one predominating sound. Thus, it is by no means uncommon to be able to discern two, or even three, main sounds in the voice.

In general, a loud voice indicates the presence of a Full condition, whereas a quiet one reflects an Empty condition. In the same way, breathing which sounds feeble and faint points to an Empty condition. A wheezing sound reflects the presence of Dampness or Phlegm in the Lungs.

The Odour The odour is more difficult than the voice to diagnose in the context of Shiatsu Therapy, simply because the receiver remains clothed. However, practitioners who train their nose will still be able to smell the natural odour of a clothed person. This odour should not be confused with the body odour produced by perspiration. It is more subtle and is most present around the chest and upper back.

A putrid, stagnant odour indicates a Kidney disharmony. A rancid, sour odour indicates a Liver imbalance (or Retention of Food). A faint scorched smell, like freshly ironed linen, points to either a Heart disharmony or the presence of Heat. A sickly sweet or 'Fragrant' odour reflects a problem with the Spleen. A rotten, musty odour indicates either a Lung disharmony or the presence of Phlegm in the body.

SOUND AND ODOUR: FIVE ELEMENT RELATIONSHIPS

	Water/ Kidney	Wood/ Liver	Fire/ Heart	Earth/ Spleen	Metal/ Lung
Sound	Groan	Shout/ clipped	Laugh/ tremulous	Sing	Weep
Odour	Putrid	Rancid	Scorched	Sweet/ Fragrant	Rotten/ musty

Chapter 20

Pulse Diagnosis

Reading the pulse according to Oriental Medicine provides information about the patient's entire constitution and condition. It accurately reflects the state of the Ki, the Blood, of Yin and Yang in the body, and of the internal Organs. Along with tongue diagnosis, it has traditionally been the most important tool of health assessment.

Pulse diagnosis in its complete form is very complex, some of which is not applicable in Shiatsu practice. What we will present here is a simplified approach.

Like Hara diagnosis, pulse diagnosis is relatively more subjective than other forms of diagnosis. It requires considerable skill in discerning the subtle distinctions between different types of pulse. Even the simple form outlined below will require additional supervised instruction and a great deal of practice to master. It should also be remembered that pulse diagnosis is often subject to short-term influences which may obscure an accurate reading of the patient's true underlying condition. Temporary states of depletion and emotional upset will be reflected in the pulse.

METHOD OF PULSE-TAKING

Ensure that the patient's arm is horizontal. It should not be held at a level higher than that of the heart. The practitioner should use their first three fingers to feel the patient's pulse, which is located along the radial artery just below the wrist.

The left-hand pulse is generally more indicative of the state of the patient's Blood. It is usually slightly stronger in men. The right-hand pulse is generally more indicative of the patient's Ki, and is usually slightly stronger in women.

A pulse which is 'gentle' and resilient and lacks any feeling of roughness indicates strong Stomach Ki. As the first Organ of digestion, the Stomach is the origin of Ki, Blood and Body Fluids, and therefore representative of the Ki as a whole. A pulse which is regular, neither strong nor weak, and maintains a consistent quality is said to have

Fig. 20.1: Pulse-taking

'spirit', and reflects a healthy condition of the Heart, Blood and Mind.

A pulse which can be clearly felt at a deep level is considered to have 'root', and reflects the condition of the Kidneys and Essence.

12 MAIN PULSE QUALITIES

1. Superficial/Floating Pulse

To feel this pulse the practitioner need only place their fingers lightly on the patient's artery.

- Indicates an External condition, as Ki rises to the surface to defend the Interior;
  Superficial and Tight: External Wind-Cold;
  Superficial and Wiry: External Wind-Heat.
- A pulse which is both Superficial and Empty at a deep level indicates Yin deficiency.

2. Deep Pulse

This pulse is opposite to a Superficial pulse and requires a deep pressure to reach it.

- Indicates an Internal condition, one that mainly involves the Yin Organs.

3. Slow Pulse

The normal rate of the pulse varies according to age and constitutional type. The following table gives rough approximations of a norm:

Age (in years)	Rate (beats per min)
1–4	90 plus
4–10	84
10–16	78
16–35	74
35–50	70
50 and over	68

A rate which is 10–20 beats slower than those indicated in the table may be considered a Slow pulse.

- A Slow pulse indicates the presence of Cold;
  Slow and Empty: indicates Cold generated from Yang deficiency;
  Slow and Full: indicates Cold of an Excess nature, usually the result of external invasion.

4. Rapid Pulse

A pulse which is 10–20 beats faster than the normal rates indicated in the table may be considered a Rapid pulse.

- A Rapid pulse indicates the presence of Heat;
  Rapid and Empty: indicates Heat generated from Yin deficiency;
  Rapid and Full: indicates Heat of an Excess nature.

5. Empty Pulse

This pulse may feel big but has no strength to it; it is soft to the touch.

- Indicates Ki-deficiency.

6. Full Pulse

This pulse feels big, full and relatively hard.

- Indicates a Full condition;
  Full and Rapid: indicates Excess Heat;
  Full and Slow: indicates Excess Cold.

7. Slippery Pulse

This pulse feels very smooth and slippery, and feels like something sliding through oil.

- Usually indicates Dampness, Phlegm or Retention of Food; can also reflect pregnancy.

8. Choppy Pulse   This pulse feels slightly rough to the touch, like a toothbrush. It can also mean a pulse which changes frequently in rate and quality.

- Indicates Blood deficiency and occasionally depletion of Body Fluids.

9. Thready/Fine/ Thin Pulse   This pulse is very fine, like a piece of thread.

- Indicates Blood deficiency and occasionally Dampness with Ki-deficiency.

10. Tight Pulse   This pulse feels hard and taut, like a twisted rope.

- Indicates a Cold condition;
  Tight and Superficial: indicates External Cold;
  Tight and Deep: indicates Internal Cold.
- A Tight pulse may also reflect pain.

11. Wiry Pulse   This pulse is thinner, harder and more taut than the Tight pulse. It is often likened to a guitar string.

- Usually indicates Liver-Ki stagnation; can also reflect pain or the presence of Phlegm.

12. Weak Pulse   This pulse is both deep and soft.

- Indicates Yang deficiency.

Chapter 21

Tongue Diagnosis

Tongue diagnosis is a very accurate and reliable way of assessing the patient's condition. It is less subjective than pulse diagnosis, may be mastered more quickly, and is generally not subject to temporary changes in the patient's condition.

It is important to have an adequate amount of natural light to see the tongue properly for detailed diagnosis. When this is not available, a small torch should be used. The patient should not have taken food or drink in the half-hour prior to observation of the tongue.

THE SHAPE OF THE TONGUE BODY

- Thin and pale: Blood deficiency   **Thin**
- Thin and red: Yin deficiency

- Swollen and pale: Spleen and/or Kidney Yang deficiency causing   **Swollen**
  Dampness
- Swollen and red: Damp Heat

- Spleen Ki deficiency   **Teeth marks around edge**

- Heat in the Heart   **Long**

- Short and pale: Spleen Yang deficiency causing Internal Cold   **Short**
- Short and red: Yin deficiency or Excess Heat

- Cracks generally indicate Yin deficiency or Excess Heat   **Cracked**
- Short horizontal cracks: Yin deficiency

Fig. 21.1: Tongue areas

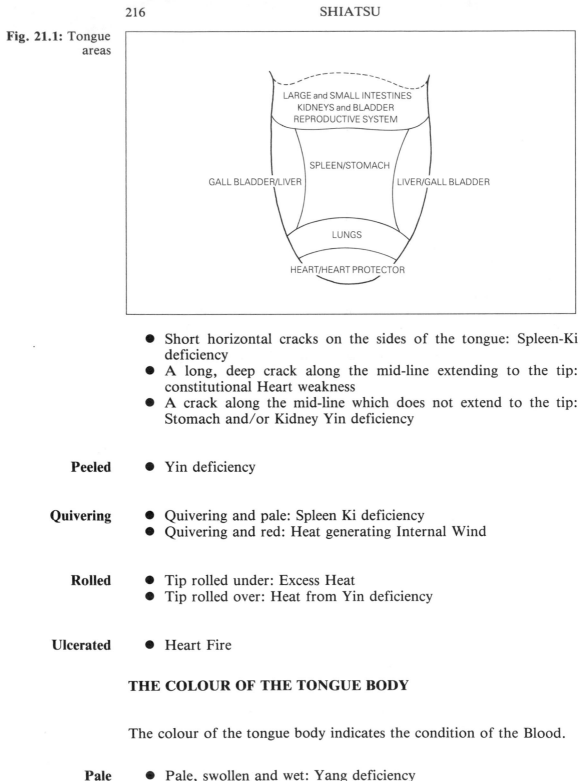

- Short horizontal cracks on the sides of the tongue: Spleen-Ki deficiency
- A long, deep crack along the mid-line extending to the tip: constitutional Heart weakness
- A crack along the mid-line which does not extend to the tip: Stomach and/or Kidney Yin deficiency

Peeled

- Yin deficiency

Quivering

- Quivering and pale: Spleen Ki deficiency
- Quivering and red: Heat generating Internal Wind

Rolled

- Tip rolled under: Excess Heat
- Tip rolled over: Heat from Yin deficiency

Ulcerated

- Heart Fire

THE COLOUR OF THE TONGUE BODY

The colour of the tongue body indicates the condition of the Blood.

Pale

- Pale, swollen and wet: Yang deficiency
- Pale and dry: Blood deficiency

- Red: Heat **Red**
- Red, dry and without coating: Heat from Yin deficiency
- Red and wet: Heat and Dampness
- Red and shiny: Stomach and/or Kidney Yin deficiency
- Scarlet red: Lung and/or Heart Yin deficiency
- Red spots: localized Heat
- Red with large red spots: Heat with stagnant Blood

- Purple: stagnation of Ki or Blood **Purple**
- Reddish purple: Ki/Blood stagnation with Heat
- Bluish-purple: Ki/Blood stagnation with Cold

- Internal Cold **Blue**

TONGUE COATING

Whereas the shape and colour of the tongue body more commonly reflect the condition of the Blood and Yin Organs, the tongue coating is particularly indicative of the state of the Yang organs, especially the Stomach.

It is in fact the Stomach which produces the tongue coating. A certain amount of Dampness is left over from the digestion of food, and travels upwards to the tongue. It is therefore normal to have a thin, white coating.

A tongue coating which is thicker than normal indicates the presence of an Internal or External pathogenic factor. An absence of tongue coating indicates Yin deficiency.

- Cold and Dampness in the Middle Heater **White and Thick**

- Normal body colour: External Wind-Cold **White, Thick and**
- Pale body colour: Internal Cold and Dampness **Wet**

- Retention of Food from Yang deficiency **White, Thick and Greasy**

- External Wind-Heat **Thin Yellow**

- Internal Damp-Heat **Thick Yellow**

Dirty Yellow   ● Damp-Heat in the Stomach and Intestines

Yellow, Sticky or   ● Phlegm-Heat
Greasy

Grey and Wet   ● Cold-Damp in the Spleen

Grey and Dry   ● Excess Heat

Chapter 22

Questioning and Case-Taking

Asking relevant questions gives a general impression of the history and lifestyle of the recipient, as well as information about the level of health or disease amongst blood relations. This information will help us to determine the underlying cause of their disharmony and will often indicate their prognosis.

For example, if a 40-year-old man presents with symptoms which suggest heart problems, and questions reveal that his father, grandfather and brother all died from heart failure before they reached the age of 45, then a major hereditary or familial problem is indicated. A poor prognosis suggests itself unless a common factor which can be treated is identified. It may be that the whole family has always subsisted on fried eggs and sugar, with a total aversion to exercise. The treatment aim is then obvious, but he may not have given this information had you not asked.

The answers to your questions, along with your observations on all levels as described throughout this chapter, will constitute the framework for a case history. Not all questions need to be answered in every case, and others may need to be added. The most important consideration is to 'communicate' with your clients, rather than interrogate them.

Of course, by simply finding and treating the most Kyo and Jitsu Channels, the energetic distortions can be positively affected. However, the case history questionnaire enables us to find out from which level of pathology the distortions arise. This means that we can assess the root cause and prognosis, and offer supplementary advice on such things as exercise, diet and lifestyle where applicable.

A CASE HISTORY FORMAT

Name: D.o.b.   Date:
Address: Male/Female:
Tel: Day: Evening:

Subjective Assessment (verbal information given by the client)

Reasons for seeking treatment
This usually reflects the symptoms most urgently in need of attention from the recipient's perspective.

Medical history
This may provide a clue to current symptoms; operations or accident trauma may have weakened or obstructed certain Channels due to the removal of organs or the build up of scar tissue, therefore causing pain local to the scar tissue, or elsewhere along the affected Channel.

The medical history may also indicate how chronic a condition is. If the client comes to be treated for eczema and questioning reveals they were born with it, and have been extensively treated using many different approaches from birth onwards, then we can conclude that it is very chronic and deep seated, and requires extensive treatment to alleviate.

Medical history of family
Include parents, grandparents, brothers and sisters. This may highlight a hereditary influence or a familial pattern such as described in the introduction to this chapter.

Medication
Past: Medical drugs may produce side effects which confuse
               the diagnosis or produce more extreme reactions to
               treatment.

Fatigue patterns
Feeling drowsy after meals indicates Spleen-Ki deficiency.
Extreme lethargy with a feeling of cold is characteristic of Kidney-Yang deficiency.

Sleep patterns
Any problems relating to sleep can result from excess Yang, Yin deficiency or Blood deficiency. However, difficulty in getting to sleep is usually due to excess Yang.

Light sleep when one wakes at the slightest sound is more often due to Blood deficiency.
Restless, disturbed sleep relates to Yin deficiency.

Hot/cold
Coldness indicates Yang deficiency.
Feeling hot can result from either excess Yang or Yin deficiency.
Heat from Yin Deficiency is more common at night and in the late afternoon.

Perspiration
Excessive perspiration can result from both excess Yang and Yin deficiency.
Yin deficiency more commonly causes sweating at night only.
Lack of perspiration may indicate deficient Yang or Cold.

Thirst
Hot conditions are characterized by the desire to drink cold liquids, usually in large volumes.
Cold conditions are characterized by a lack of thirst or the desire to drink warm liquids; usually the Stomach or Spleen is implicated.

Diet and digestion
Empty conditions are usually relieved by eating.
Full conditions are usually aggravated by eating.
Lack of appetite reflects Spleen Ki deficiency.
Constant hunger reflects Heat in the Stomach.
Distension after eating indicates Retention of Food.
Hot conditions create a craving for Cold food.
Cold conditions create a craving for Hot food.
Food fads and extreme dietary philosophies may encourage an inappropriate diet for the individual, often generating symptoms of deficiency.

Alcohol
Excessive alcohol consumption tends to generate Heat in the body and deplete the Yin. It may also give rise to disharmonies of the Liver.

Smoking
Smoking leads to the creation of Heat and Phlegm in the Lungs and Heart. This can lead to lung cancer and heart disease. In our experience, because smoking produces Heat in the Blood, skin problems cannot be resolved until the client ceases to smoke.

Drugs

The majority of 'recreational' drugs are extremely deleterious to the bodymind and seriously injure the Ki, Blood and Essence.

Prolonged use of drugs such as heroin and cocaine generates Heat, consumes the Yin of the Kidneys, Stomach and Heart, and causes Liver-Ki stagnation.

Hallucinogenic drugs and amphetamines particularly weaken the nervous system.

All such drugs disturb the Mind (Shen) and can lead to depression, anxiety, paranoia and aggressive behaviour.

Pain

The assessment of pain is very useful in Shiatsu because it reflects directly the circulation and quantity of Ki in the channels, which can be directly or indirectly influenced by Shiatsu. If the Channels are free from obstruction there is no pain.

Sharp, localized pain, as in Jitsu conditions, can be caused by:

- invasion by external pathogenic factors
- stagnation of Ki, Blood or Phlegm
- obstruction by Phlegm   obstructing Ki in
- retention of Food   the Channels
- internal Cold or Heat

Dull, empty, less focused pain reflects deficiency conditions, or Kyo within the Channels. It is caused by deficiency of Ki and Blood.

Headaches

The most common type of headache is caused by stress and feels 'tight', like a band around the head, or from the back of the neck towards the eyes. This results from Liver-Ki stagnation and is also often accompanied by nausea.

Another common type of headache is a pounding or throbbing type, often accompanied by a burning sensation in the eyes. This is caused by Liver-Yang rising or Liver-Fire.

Headaches with a deep, boring pain result from Blood deficiency or Blood stagnation.

Headaches on the front of the head are commonly caused by Stomach problems, e.g. Retention of Food, often accompanied by indigestion.

Headaches on the back of the head often involve the Kidneys.

Menstruation

Pre-menstrual tension and pre-menstrual pain both result from stagnation of Liver Ki or Blood.

Pain during the period is usually caused by Heat in the Blood or stagnation of Cold.

Pain and weakness after the period is caused by Blood deficiency.
Heavy periods when the Blood is dark red or bright are caused by
Heat in the Blood.
Heavy bleeding when the Blood is pale is caused by Ki deficiency.
Scanty Blood or absence of menstruation is caused by Blood
deficiency or stagnation of Blood.
Clots in the menstrual Blood indicate stagnation of Blood.

Bowels

Constipation may be caused by Liver-Ki stagnation, Blood
deficiency, Yin deficiency, or Heat.
Loose stools and diarrhoea generally suggest Spleen-Yang or Kidney-
Yang deficiency.
Alternating constipation and diarrhoea are typical of Liver Ki
invading the Spleen.

Urine

Scanty urination indicates Kidney-Yin deficiency.
Large amounts of pale urine indicate Kidney-Yang deficiency.
Pale urine indicates Cold conditions whereas dark urine indicates
Heat.

Objective Assessment (Information you acquire using your
senses: seeing, hearing, smelling, touching)

Skin

Skin conditions often point to a condition of the Lungs. However,
the following factors can also affect the skin: Heat in the Blood
caused by Liver or Stomach Heat; stagnation or deficiency of Liver
Blood. These conditions cause dryness, redness, itching and scaling
skin. Pus conditions involve Dampness or Phlegm.

Swellings

All abnormal lumps should be checked by a medical doctor if they
have not previously been examined, especially if they look or feel
like cauliflower, or are growing or changing in any way.
Pitting oedema, called water oedema in Chinese Medicine, results
from Kidney Yang deficiency.

Posture

A general sense of strength or weakness, rigidity or openness,
depression or optimism, can be observed in the posture.
Differences in the height of each shoulder, or other anomalies are
worth checking as they may indicate some distortions in the Channels
or skeletal structure. Such distortions may be the cause or the result
of dysfunctions within the internal organs.

Constitutional type
See p.191.

Breathing
Shallow breathing can indicate Lung-Ki deficiency.
Wheezing can mean Phlegm in the Lungs.
Constriction in the chest can arise because of Liver Ki stagnation.

Nails
See p.197.

Face
See p.194.

Tongue
See p.215.

Pulse
See p.211.

Hara
See p.201.

Back
See p.199.

Element Correspondences

- **Colour**   (see page 194)
- **Sound**
- **Odour**   (see page 210)
- **Emotion**

Comments
Any other information considered relevant, such as stiffness in specific joints, general attitude of the client, and so on, should be included.

Conclusion (Diagnosis)

A common thread will emerge from the case history which will substantiate the Hara, Back or Pulse diagnosis. Experience gives the practitioner the ability to extract what is relevant, and to narrow down all the presenting factors to reveal the underlying causes of the recipient's condition.

Chapter 23

Case Study Examples

CASE No. 1: KIDNEY KYO/LUNG JITSU

A woman in her early fifties comes for treatment complaining of mild asthma, a 'wheezy' chest and difficulty in catching her breath. Further questioning reveals that she is often tired, feels cold and has copious, clear urination. Her pulse is Empty and her tongue pale and slightly swollen.

In terms of Traditional Oriental Medicine, this is an example of the Kidneys failing to grasp Ki from the Lungs. It is confirmed by a Jitsu condition of the Lung Channel together with a Kyo condition of the Kidney Channel.

The client's asthma, chest congestion and difficulty in catching her breath result from a failure of the Lungs to fulfil their function of descending the Ki. As a result, excess Ki accumulates in the Upper Heater to produce what appears to be a Full condition of the Lungs. It is this apparently Full condition which leads to the Jitsu quality of the Lung Channel.

Part of this condition, however, is a failure of the Kidneys to grasp Ki from the Lungs – a problem which arises from Kidney-Yang deficiency. Deficient Kidney-Yang is evident from her tiredness, feelings of cold and copious, clear urination. The Empty pulse and pale, swollen tongue further confirm a Yang deficient condition.

Treatment Tonifying the Kidney Channel and Tsubos such as Bladder-23 may in itself be enough to rectify this basically Deficient situation. However, dispersal of the Lung Channel may be necessary if the chest is especially congested with Phlegm.
(For details of treating Kidney-Lung disharmony see p.150.)

CASE No. 2: KIDNEY KYO/LIVER JITSU

A man in his early forties comes for treatment complaining of lower back pain, insomnia, frequent headaches and sore, inflamed eyes.

Further questioning reveals that he is frequently thirsty and sweats profusely at night. You notice that he is restless and irritable. His pulse has a Floating quality. His tongue is red, has no coating, is peeled at the rear and swollen at the sides.

In terms of Traditional Oriental Medicine, this is an example of a combination of Kidney-Yin deficiency and Liver-Yang rising. It is confirmed by the fact that the Kidney Channel presents as Kyo in condition and the Liver Channel as Jitsu.

Kidney deficiency is evident from the lower back pain. The patient's thirst, night sweats, insomnia and restlessness are clear indicators of Yin-deficiency. Yin-deficiency is also apparent from a red, peeled tongue without coating. The Kidney-Yin is clearly failing to nourish the Liver-Yin and so 'hold down' the Liver-Yang.

The consequent rising Liver-Yang has resulted in headaches, eye inflammation and irritability. Swelling along the sides of the tongue indicates a Full condition of the Liver. A Floating pulse reveals that the body's Yang has risen to the surface because of a depletion of Yin.

Treatment This is an example of how Yin/Yang disharmony in the body can create a basically Kyo condition underlying signs of Jitsu. The Excess Yang/Jitsu condition of the Liver stems directly from the deficient Yin/Kyo condition of the Kidney. The priority in treatment, therefore, is to tonify the Kidney Kyo, and so 'bring down' the Liver Jitsu. It may, however, be necessary to disperse the Liver Channel if the patient is suffering acute symptoms (such as headache) caused by Liver Jitsu. (For details of treating Kidney-Yin deficiency, see p.149; for Liver-Yang rising, see p.156.)

CASE No. 3: LIVER JITSU/SPLEEN KYO

A man in his late twenties comes for treatment complaining of abdominal discomfort, flatulence and alternating periods of constipation and diarrhoea. He reports that he feels tired 'most of the time'. You also notice that he is tense, and indeed, he says he thinks that his problems are related to stress. His tongue is generally pale but red on the sides.

This is a clear example of the 'Liver invading the Spleen'. Stagnant Liver-Ki can readily affect the Spleen if the Spleen-Ki or Spleen-Yang are weak. Wood 'invades' Earth along the Control Cycle of the Five Elements, thus impeding the transformative function of the Spleen.

Stagnant Liver-Ki is indicated by symptoms of a 'stuck' digestion, tension, and redness on the sides of the tongue. It is a Full condition which gives a Jitsu quality to the Liver channel.

Because stagnant Ki is actively weakening Spleen-Yang, the patient feels tired and has a pale tongue. That the Spleen's transformative function is impaired is apparent from the patient's flatulence and **Treatment** diarrhoea. The Spleen's condition is Empty, and is reflected in the Kyo quality of its Channel.

Finally, the patient's constipation is primarily the result of stagnant Liver-Ki; the fact that it alternates with diarrhoea is an obvious indication of Liver-Spleen disharmony.

It is necessary in this situation both to invigorate the stagnant Liver-Ki and reinforce Spleen-Yang. One must therefore disperse the Jitsu condition of the Liver Channel as well as tonify the Kyo of the Spleen. Stimulation of Tsubos such as Gall Bladder-34 and Spleen-6 will support this treatment.

Very often, however, there will be a predominance of symptoms relating either to the Liver Jitsu or the Spleen Kyo. If stagnant Liver-Ki predominates the patient will obviously exhibit a 'stuck' condition, reporting a greater degree of tension and constipation. If the deficient Spleen-Yang is a greater problem the patient will be largely Kyo in condition, complaining more of tiredness and diarrhoea. The practitioner may therefore need to place a stronger emphasis on either tonification or dispersal, depending on the patient's predominant condition.

(For details of treating Spleen deficiency, see p.168; Stagnation of Liver-Ki, see p.154.)

CASE No. 4: HEART JITSU/LUNG KYO

A woman in her late fifties comes for treatment complaining of occasional palpitations, a feeling of oppression and fullness in the chest, breathlessness and a lack of energy. Upon further questioning you learn that several months ago she visited her doctor after experiencing some pains in the chest. Her face is a bright pale colour, her lips are slightly blue and her hands are cold. She also mentions that she is prone to sweating in the day for no apparent reason. Her pulse is Empty; her tongue pale and slightly purple.

In terms of Oriental Medicine, the patient's condition combines an apparently Full pattern of the Heart (stagnation of Heart-Blood), with an Empty pattern of the Lungs (Lung-Ki deficiency). However, the underlying condition of the Heart is one of deficiency, producing a situation that calls for careful application of tonification and dispersal.

Symptoms of stagnant Heart-Blood include palpitations, feelings of oppression and fullness in the chest, and chest pain. Cold hands, bluish lips and a slightly purple tongue are further indications of an impeded blood circulation. Although this condition creates signs and symptoms characterized by Fullness, it has arisen because of a failure of the Yang to transport and circulate blood.

That there is an underlying Ki- and Yang-deficient condition is made particularly apparent by the Ki-deficient condition of the Lungs. This pattern is manifesting in the patient through her breathlessness, tiredness, pallor and sweating during the day. This last symptom is a result of a weakness in the body's Defensive Ki (controlled by the Lungs) in regulating the pores of the skin. When Lung-Ki is weak the pores lose their tone and allow sweat to leak out spontaneously. Deficient Lung-Ki is further evident in the patient's Empty pulse and generally pale tongue.

It is clear that two patterns indicated here – that of stagnant Heart-Blood and Lung-Ki deficiency – are closely connected, and are both associated with a weakness of Gathering (or Chest) Ki. Gathering Ki provides both Organs with their motive force. Although the Heart Channel exhibits a Jitsu quality reflecting a degree of stasis, the underlying condition of the Organ is deficient. The Kyo Lung Channel more accurately reflects a basically deficient situation.

Treatment It is necessary in this instance to tonify the Ki and Yang of the Heart and Lungs without failing to assist the movement of Blood in the chest. Treatment should commence with an emphasis on tonifying Kyo, especially along the Lung Channel and in the chest. Tonification of the Tsubos Bladder-13, Directing Vessel-17 and Lung-9 will support this process. If the Heart Channel remains Jitsu in condition, gently disperse the Heart and possibly Heart Protector Channels (including Tsubos such as Heart Protector-6). This will help to regulate the flow of Blood in the chest.

(For details of treating Stagnation of Heart-Blood, see p.163, for Lung-Ki deficiency, see p.173.)

PART 4

CONCLUSIONS

Chapter 24

The Five Elements and Hara Focus

The general principles of Oriental Medicine as applied to Shiatsu therapy have been presented in the previous sections. In this chapter we have condensed and translated the essential aspects of each of the Five Elements in order to directly influence treatment. We do this by ascribing to each Element a particular energetic and mental focus. Each energetic technique and associated Hara focus is based on the primary functions and faculties extracted from their corresponding Element.

All the energetic techniques and qualities of Hara presented are essential to good Shiatsu. However, the ability to emphasize a particular quality of Ki, either through visualization or inner sensory focus, will give the practitioner an opportunity to create a specific effect. The effect chosen will be determined by the nature of the recipient's condition.

For example, bodily and psychological symptoms which result from a deficiency of Earth will require an emphasis on support, ultimately enhanced by projecting a nurturing quality from the Hara.

Key words which indicate the nuance of each Element are displayed in italics within the summary of each Element given below. These key words are subsequently compared in the form of a table at the end of this chapter.

WATER

The Water Element represents the origin of life, *conception*. One of its associated functions is to ensure survival. On a biological level, it achieves this through *procreation*, facilitated in part by interaction, a function of the preceding Element of Metal. These functions are part of the faculty of *Will* and are supported by our innate *drive*.

The effect of Will and drive upon Ki is both to *concentrate* it and provide the *motive force* behind the functions of the Organs. The Kidneys concentrate the Ki in the sense that they are responsible for the formation of Essence, which is Ki at its most condensed and consolidated. The motivating power of Water is clearly apparent in the action of the Original Ki, which promotes the transformation of Ki at every stage of its formation (see p.128).

These energetic activities are best encouraged in Shiatsu through an emphasis on *holding techniques*. Holding techniques attract and concentrate Ki, and in so doing, tonify the motive force behind Organ function. The *concentration of Ki* will be promoted by a *one-pointed focus* on the root of the Hara at Tanden (located at the Tsubo Directing Vessel-6).

WOOD

The procreation of repeated generations progresses in such a way as to ensure the continual *adaptation and growth* of the species. This is the process of *evolution*, a function associated with Wood. On a personal psychological level, evolution expresses itself as a desire to expand the limits of one's being. This desire is the result of aspiration and *vision*, qualities which are dependent upon having a sense of *direction* in life. They naturally arise when the Liver ensures that the flow of Ki is *smooth*. Ki which is obstructed and stagnates blocks a sense of direction and therefore frustrates growth.

In order to enhance these aspects of the Wood Element, the emphasis during treatment should be on the *smoothing and 'opening'* of Ki. To promote the 'opening' of stiff and aching musculature and move stagnant Ki, a *relaxed and open Hara* is essential.

FIRE

Personal evolution and growth lead to *realization*, a function associated with the Fire Element. Realization can only come through constant *self-reflection* and *unconditional love*, and is the ultimate purpose of *consciousness*. The power of a clear and accepting awareness lies in the ability to *harmonize* the conflicting thoughts and emotions that sometimes arise within.

Consciousness *expands and rarefies Ki* and resides in the Heart as the Shen (or the Mind). The Shen embraces in its function every possible mental activity within the individual. Because the Shen is the most sensitive aspect of the bodymind, easily affected by both emotional and physical disharmonies, it is vital for the practitioner to develop the ability to *harmonize and calm*. This treatment emphasis will naturally manifest if the practitioner radiates a feeling of *empathy* from the Heart, while at the same time remaining anchored in the Hara. This energetic stance reflects the function of the Kidneys in anchoring the Shen.

EARTH

Once realization has been achieved, the next stage is to take the ideals of Fire and make them reality. This is the role of the Earth Element: that of *actualization (and materialization)*. Life on a material level is supported by the process of *nourishment*, the central function of the Spleen and Stomach. As well as being responsible for the digestion and *absorption* of food, Earth also provides the capacity to digest ideas and information. It *transforms* food into Blood and mental stimuli into *Thought*, and therefore nourishes both body and Mind.

The role of Earth is primarily one of providing sustenance and *support*. It can thus be strengthened through Shiatsu treatment which itself places an emphasis on *support*. A nurturing quality of touch will most naturally manifest when the Hara is experienced as a *stable ground*.

METAL

Once the Self has been consolidated in material form there is a need to reach beyond the limits of one's physical shell and make contact with the environment. Our urge to *interact* with others and *participate* in the world around us finds an outlet through the ability to *communicate*. The Metal Element is the sensitive surface or the 'skin' with which we touch and feel, communicate and receive.

Making energetic and psychological contact with our surroundings maintains our *vitality*. This is most clearly seen at work on a biological level in the process of respiration, through which energy is continually *exchanged and renewed*. This function in the human body is dominated by the Lungs, the Organ which governs the Ki. Through the Lungs, the Metal Element therefore *revitalizes and disseminates energy*. It ensures a vitality of Spirit through the dynamic involvement of the individual with their environment.

The Metal Element's functions of communication and energy exchange most directly relate to Shiatsu treatment which places an emphasis on *connection* with the recipient. A strong communication ensures two important things: the maximum *projection of Ki* from practitioner to recipient; and a feeling of mutual interaction. The quality of Hara which best encourages connection is therefore one of *projecting Ki*.

	Water	Wood	Fire	Earth	Metal
Associated functions	conception	evolution	realization	materialization, actualization	participation interaction
	procreation and survival	growth and adaptation	love and self-reflection	nourishment	communication
Faculty	Will	vision	consciousness	Thought	vitality
Power	drive	direction	harmonization	absorption	energy exchange/renewal
Effect upon Ki	concentrates and motivates	smoothes	expands and rarefies	transforms	vitalizes and disseminates
Treatment emphasis	holding	smoothing, 'opening'	harmonizing, calming	supporting	connecting
Hara Focus	concentrated, one-pointed	relaxed and open	empathizing	stable ground	projecting

Chapter 25

The Value of Shiatsu

Shiatsu given with a genuine desire to help others becomes in itself an avenue for personal growth and development.

An integral part of any growth in consciousness involves developing a greater sense of compassion for all living beings. Empathy to realize when and to what extent another being is suffering, together with the motivation to relieve suffering, are the basic requirements for practising any method of healing. Shiatsu helps to foster empathy through touch. It calls for motivation which is free from the constraints of the ego and its in-built limitations.

The motivation to help alleviate suffering requires discipline in order to gain the necessary skills, for such skills are born of careful study and self-reflection. By centring the Mind and strengthening the Hara, by finding the stable ground within, discipline comes naturally. Only then can we discover our true potential.

Discipline expresses itself as constant practice, allowing knowledge to sink deeper and deeper with each Shiatsu treatment we give. Practice can also mean spiritual practice and other ways of deepening ourselves. Study, self-reflection and practice all work together to make a good practitioner. Only by helping ourselves can we be of value to others.

Shiatsu enhances the lives of both giver and receiver, employing and revivifying the feeling of connectedness in the two. As givers we become fitter, more flexible, more open and centred, having found the well of our vital source. Through our intimate appreciation of the interplay of Ki we become more connected to all of life around us.

Appendix

GLOSSARY OF TSUBOS

Bladder Channel

Bladder-2
In the hollow on the medial side of the eyebrow, in the supraorbital notch.
- Benefits the eyes. May be used as a local Tsubo for any problem affecting the eyes, especially when the Liver is involved.
- Eases pain in the face by eliminating obstruction and Wind along the Channel of the face; useful in cases of frontal headaches and hay fever.

Bladder-10
At the base of the occipital bone, 1.3 cun* lateral to the posterior median line.
- Alleviates occipital headache, neck stiffness and nasal congestion caused by an invasion of External Wind-Cold.
- Subdues the rising of Internal Liver-Wind which causes dizziness, vertigo and occipital headache.
- Stimulates the brain, enhances concentration and benefits the eyes, especially when there is Kidney deficiency.

Bladder-11
Gathering Point for the Bones
Sea of Blood Point
1.5 cun lateral to the lower end of the spinous process of the 1st thoracic vertebra.

- Strengthens the bones, e.g. in cases of chronic arthritis and osteoporosis.
- Nourishes the Blood in cases of rheumatic muscular pain, especially when it 'wanders' around the body.

* A 'cun' is a unit of measurement used in Oriental Medicine which is approximately equivalent to the recipient's thumb at its widest part. It is sometimes referred to as an 'anatomical Chinese inch' (ACI).

- Expels External Wind in a similar way to Bladder-12, though not as strongly.

Bladder-12
1.5 cun lateral to the lower end of the spinous process of the 2nd thoracic vertebra.

- Disperses External Wind: relieves the symptoms of colds and influenza; can also be used to prevent the invasion of External Wind.
- Regulates Lung-Ki.

Bladder-13
Transporting (Yu) Point of the Lungs
1.5 cun lateral to the lower end of the spinous process of the 3rd thoracic vertebra.

- Promotes the descending and dispersing function of the Lungs; disperses External Wind and relieves coughs and asthma.
- Tonifies Lung-Ki; useful in cases of dyspnoea, lethargy and melancholy.
- Tonifies Lung-Yin; may be used for Heat in the chest.

Bladder-14
Transporting (Yu) Point of the Heart Protector
1.5 cun lateral to the lower end of the spinous process of the 4th thoracic vertebra.

- Regulates the function of the Heart and Pericardium; useful in cases of palpitations, irregular heartbeat and pericarditis.
- Uplifts and calms the Mind.
- Benefits the teeth and gums; may be used for inflammatory disorders of the dental nerves.

Bladder-15
Transporting (Yu) Point of the Heart
1.5 cun lateral to the lower end of the spinous process of the 5th thoracic vertebra.

- Calms the Mind and clears Heat when the Heart is agitated; may be used for problems such as anxiety, restlessness and insomnia.
- Moves the Blood in the chest region; relieves angina pectoris.
- Enhances powers of concentration; strengthens memory.

Bladder-17
Transporting (Yu) Point for the Diaphragm
Gathering Point for the Blood
1.5 cun lateral to the lower end of the spinous process of the 7th thoracic vertebra.

- Moves the Blood; may be used for Blood stagnation anywhere in the body.
- Nourishes the Blood; useful in cases of dizziness, blurred vision and lethargy due to Blood deficiency; use moxibustion.

- Relieves tension and spasm in the diaphragm which causes indigestion and a bloated sensation.

Bladder-18
Transporting (Yu) Point for the Liver
1.5 cun lateral to the lower end of the spinous process of the 9th thoracic vertebra.
- Benefits the Liver and Gall Bladder, especially when they are affected either by Ki stagnation (causing nausea, pain under the ribs and irritability) or Damp-Heat (causing jaundice).
- Tonifies Liver-Blood and nourishes the eyes.

Bladder-19
Transporting (Yu) Point for the Gall Bladder
1.5 cun lateral to the lower end of the spinous process of the 10th thoracic vertebra.
- Clears Heat and Damp-Heat in the Liver and Gall Bladder; useful in cases of hepatitis.
- Regulates Stomach-Ki; often useful for relieving belching and acid reflux ('heartburn').
- Relaxes the diaphragm.

Bladder-20
Transporting (Yu) Point for the Spleen
1.5 cun lateral to the lower end of the spinous process of the 11th thoracic vertebra.
- Strengthens the Spleen and Stomach; useful in cases of tiredness, poor digestion and loose stools.
- Clears Dampness due to an impairment of the Spleen's transformative and transportative functions; useful in cases of excessive catarrh production and oedema in the torso.
- Promotes the Spleen's formation of Blood; may be used in cases of anaemia; use moxibustion.

Bladder-21
Transporting (Yu) Point for the Stomach
1.5 cun lateral to the lower end of the spinous process of the 12th thoracic vertebra.
- Strengthens the Stomach and Spleen; useful for weakness of Ki and Blood due to Stomach and Spleen deficiency; clears Dampness.
- Promotes the descending of Stomach-Ki; relieves Food Retention, abdominal bloating and indigestion.

Bladder-22
Transporting (Yu) Point for the Triple Heater
1.5 cun lateral to the lower end of the spinous process of the 1st lumbar vertebra.
- Clears Dampness; promotes the transformation of fluids, especially in the Lower Heater; often useful in cases of oedema.

Bladder-23
Transporting (Yu) Point for the Kidneys
1.5 cun lateral to the lower end of the spinous process of the 2nd lumbar vertebra.
- Tonifies Kidney-Yang; useful in cases of general debility, excessive urination and feelings of cold; empowers the Will.
- Strengthens Kidney-Essence and the Sea of Bone Marrow; may be used for infertility and weakness of the bones; nourishes the brain.
- Promotes the action of the Kidneys in the formation of Blood.
- Helps the Kidneys to grasp the Ki from the Lungs; often useful in cases of asthma.
- Relieves chronic lower back pain.
- Treats chronic problems of the eyes and ears.

DO NOT OVER-STIMULATE IN PREGNANCY

Bladder-25
Transporting (Yu) Point for the Large Intestines
1.5 cun lateral to the lower end of the spinous process of the 4th lumbar vertebra.
- Benefits the Large Intestines; may be used to treat both constipation and diarrhoea; useful in cases of colitis.
- Alleviates lower back pain; may be used for sciatica.

Bladder-27
Transporting (Yu) Point for the Small Intestines
1.5 cun lateral to the spine, level with the 1st posterior sacral foramen.
- Benefits the Small Intestines; clears Heat and Dampness from the Small Intestines and the urinary tract; often useful in cases of abdominal distension and discomfort, diarrhoea and cystitis.

Bladder-28
Transporting (Yu) Point for the Bladder
1.5 cun lateral to the midline of the spine, level with the 2nd posterior sacral foramen.
- Benefits the Bladder; expels Dampness from the Bladder causing difficult urination; clears Heat from the Bladder causing a burning pain on urination; may be used for all urinary problems.
- Transforms fluids in the Lower Heater; often useful in cases of oedema.

Bladder-40 (sometimes known as Bladder-54)
Earth point
At the mid point of the transverse crease of the popliteal fossa, behind the knee.
- Alleviates acute lower back ache of a Full nature.
- Invigorates the Blood in the lower legs; useful in the case of varicose veins.
- Cools the Blood; may be used for heat rashes.
- Clears Damp-Heat from the Bladder.

Bladder-43 (sometimes known as Bladder-38)
The outer Bladder-line Tsubo for the Transporting Point of the Heart Protector (Bladder-14)
3 cun lateral to lower end of spinous process of the 4th thoracic vertebra.
- Strengthens the Ki of the entire body; may be used for chronic debility.
- Tonifies Lung-Yin; useful for dry cough and chronic asthma.
- Nourishes the Kidney-Essence and the brain.

Bladder-52 (sometimes known as Bladder-47)
The outer Bladder-line Tsubo for the Transporting Point of the Kidneys (Bladder-23)
3 cun lateral to the lower end of the spinous process of the 2nd lumbar vertebra.
- Tonifies the Kidneys; expecially useful for chronic lower back pain.
- Empowers the Will; reawakens a sense of determination when there is a lack of resolve.

Bladder-57
In a hollow in the middle of the calf, midway between the transverse crease at the back of the knee and the heel.
- Alleviates lower back ache with pain radiating down the legs.
- Eases muscular stiffness and tension in the lower legs; may be used for cramping in the gastrocnemius.
- Invigorates the Blood; may be used in the case of haemorrhoids and varicose veins.

Bladder-60
Fire point
In the depression midway between the lateral malleolus and the Achilles tendon.
- Alleviates chronic back ache of an Empty nature; may be used to relieve occipital headaches due to Kidney deficiency.
- Disperses External and Internal Wind, especially in the upper parts of the body; relieves rheumatic pain, stiffness and spasm in the shoulders and neck.
- Invigorates the Blood; may be used for dysmenorrhoea with clots in menstrual blood.
- Clears Heat from the Bladder.

CONTRAINDICATED IN PREGNANCY

Bladder-67
Metal point
On the little toe, 0.1 cun from the lower lateral corner of the cuticle of the toenail.
- Disperses External and Internal Wind; alleviates headache, nasal congestion and eye problems.
- Stimulates the pituitary gland.

CONTRAINDICATED IN PREGNANCY

Directing Vessel

Directing Vessel-3
Front Collecting (Bo) Point of the Bladder
4 cun directly below the navel.
- Benefits the Bladder; clears Damp-Heat from the Bladder; useful in cases of cystitis and urinary retention.
- Promotes the function of the Uterus; alleviates menstrual problems such as amenorrhoea.

CONTRAINDICATED IN PREGNANCY

Directing Vessel-4
Collecting (Bo) Point of the Small Intestines
Meeting Point of the Directing Vessel, Kidneys, Spleen and Liver
3 cun directly below the navel.
- Nourishes the Yin and Blood of the entire body; anchors and calms the Mind.
- Tonifies the Yang of the entire body, especially treated with moxibustion; useful in cases of chronic debility.
- Strengthens the Kidneys and the Original Ki.
- Promotes the function of the Uterus; regulates menstruation.
- Benefits the Small Intestines.

CONTRAINDICATED IN PREGNANCY

Directing Vessel-5
Collecting (Bo) Point of the Triple Heater
2 cun directly below the navel.
- Tonifies the Original Ki through promoting the action of the Triple Heater.
- Clears excess fluids from the Lower Heater.

CONTRAINDICATED IN PREGNANCY

Directing Vessel-6
1.5 cun directly below the navel.
- Tonifies the Ki and Yang of the entire body, especially treated with moxibustion; tonifies Kidney-Yang and Original Ki; strengthens weakness.
- Moves the Ki; useful for stagnation of Ki in the intestines and lower abdomen causing swelling and discomfort.
- Strengthens the Spleen and clears Dampness in the lower abdomen; may be used in cases of vaginal discharge.

CONTRAINDICATED IN PREGNANCY

Directing Vessel-8
In middle of the navel.
- Tonifies the Yang; may be used for extreme fatigue and Cold.
- Tonifies the Spleen-Yang; may be used for diarrhoea.

Directing Vessel-12
Collecting (Bo) Point of the Stomach and Middle Heater
Gathering Point for the Yang Organs

4 cun directly above the navel.
- Strengthens the Stomach and Spleen; good for digestive weakness, appetite loss and the accumulation of Dampness.
- Dispels Cold from the Stomach when treated with moxibustion.

Directing Vessel-14
Collecting (Bo) Point of the Heart
Beneath the sternum, 1 cun below Directing Vessel-15, and approximately 6 cun above the navel.
- Calms the Mind and pacifies the Stomach; may be used for nervous indigestion and nausea.

Directing Vessel-15
0.5 cun below the xiphoid process, 7 cun directly above the navel.
- Calms the Mind (Shen) by nourishing the Yin and Original Ki of the Yin Organs; good for anxiety, apprehension and worry.

Directing Vessel-17
Collecting (Bo) Point of the Heart Protector and Upper Heater
Gathering Point for Ki
On the sternum, half-way between and slightly above the articulations of the right and left fifth rib.
- Tonifies the Ki of the entire body by promoting the transformation of Ki in the chest.
- Moves Ki in the chest; disperses Fullness; may be used for difficult or constricted breathing and pain in the chest.
- Clears Phlegm from the Lungs; relieves cough.
- Promotes lactation of the breasts.

Gall Bladder Channel

Gall Bladder-1
0.5 cun lateral to the outer canthus of the eye.
- Clears Wind-Heat and Liver-Fire from the eyes; may be used as a local Tsubo for inflammatory eye disorders such as conjunctivitis.
- Gives local relief of headache due to Liver-Fire and Liver-Yang rising (affects the temple area).

Gall Bladder-12
Behind the ear, within the angle formed by the posterior border of the mastoid process and the inferior edge of the occipital bone.
- Relieves occipital headache and insomnia due to Liver-Fire and Liver-Yang rising.
- Eliminates both External and Internal Wind from the head.
- Alleviates toothache.

Gall Bladder-20
Between the mastoid process and the hollow below the tuberosity of the occipital bone, and between the trapezius and sternocleidomastoid muscles.

- Disperses External Wind; especially useful in cases of neck stiffness, headache and earache due to a cold or influenza.
- Eliminates Internal Wind causing dizziness and spasms.
- Sedates Liver-Yang and Liver-Fire causing occipital headaches and problems of the eyes and ears.
- Calms and clears the Mind.

Gall Bladder-21
Mid-way between the spinous process of the 7th cervical vertebra and the acromion of the shoulder.
- Moves Ki and eases muscular tension in the shoulders and neck.
- Helps expel the placenta following childbirth.
- Stimulates lactation in the nursing mother.

CONTRAINDICATED IN PREGNANCY

Gall Bladder-24
Front Collecting (Bo) Point of the Gall Bladder
In the 7th intercostal space, on the paramedian nipple line.
- Clears Damp-Heat in the Gall Bladder and Liver causing nausea, jaundice and cholecystitis.
- Smoothes the flow of Liver-Ki.

Gall Bladder-25
Front Collecting (Bo) Point of the Kidneys
On the lateral aspect of the torso, just below the end of the 12th rib.
- Tonifies Kidney-Yang and eliminates Dampness from the Lower Heater; may be used in cases of oedema, abdominal distension and difficult urination due to Kidney-Yang deficiency.

Gall Bladder-30
One-third the way along a line drawn from the greater trochanter of the femur to the sacral hiatus.
- Moves Ki and Blood in the hips and legs; eliminates painful obstructions; useful in cases of sciatica and rheumatism.
- Strengthens the waist and thighs.
- Clears Damp-Heat in the Lower Heater; may be used for itching of the anus and genitals.
- Tonifies the Ki and Blood of the entire body.

Gall Bladder-34
Earth Point
Gathering Point for the Sinews
In the hollow anterior to and slightly below the head of the fibula.
- Helps smooth the flow of Liver-Ki, especially when it 'invades' the Stomach and Spleen; descends 'rebellious Ki' in the Stomach; often useful in cases of nausea and indigestion.
- Eliminates Damp-Heat, especially in the Gall Bladder and Liver; clears Phlegm-Fire in the Stomach.
- Benefits the sinews; relaxes the tendons and muscles throughout the body; often useful in cases of rheumatism.

- Promotes the circulation of Ki and Blood in the lower extremities; strengthens the legs.

Gall Bladder-37

5 cun above the lateral malleolus of the ankle, at the anterior margin of the fibula.

- Benefits the eyes; brightens vision; clears Liver-Fire and Wind from the eyes; may be used for such problems as conjunctivitis.

Gall Bladder-39

Gathering Point for Marrow

3 cun directly above the lateral malleolus of the ankle, between the posterior margin of the fibula and the tendon of the peroneus longus muscle.

- Nourishes Kidney-Essence and Marrow; strengthens the bones and the brain; eliminates Internal Wind.
- Expels External Wind-Damp causing rheumatic pain and neck stiffness.

Gall Bladder-40

In the hollow just below and slightly anterior to the lateral malleolus of the ankle.

- Smoothes the flow of Liver-Ki; opens the Channels and relaxes the joints; may be used for pain in the neck, flanks and buttocks.

Gall Bladder-41

Wood point

In the hollow just in front of the meeting of the 4th and 5th metatarsal bones.

- Helps smooth the flow of Liver-Ki, especially in cases of headache, dysmenorrhoea and breast pain.
- Clears Damp-Heat from the genital region; often useful for cystitis and leukorrhoea.

Heart Channel

Heart-3

Water Point

In the depression between the end of the transverse crease on the ulnar side of the elbow and the medial condyle of the humerus.

- Clears Heat and Fire from the Heart and calms the Mind; often useful in cases of mental agitation and insomnia.
- Uplifts the Spirit in cases of depression.
- Eliminates painful obstructions along the Heart Channel.

Heart-5

On the ulnar aspect of the forearm, 1 cun above Heart-7.

- Tonifies Heart-Ki and calms the Mind; useful for palpitations, arrhythmia and breathlessness due to weakness of Heart-Ki.
- Benefits the tongue and promotes speech; may be used for 'stage fright'.

Heart-6
On the ulnar aspect of the forearm, 0.5 cun above Heart-7.
- Nourishes Heart-Yin and calms the Mind; useful for palpitations, anxiety, night sweating and thirst due to a deficiency of Heart-Yin.
- Stops excessive perspiration.

Heart-7
Earth Point
In the small hollow on the ulnar aspect at the end of the transverse crease of the wrist, on the proximal radial side of the pisiform bone.
- Nourishes Heart-Blood; calms and benefits the Mind; useful for anxiety, irritability, insomnia and dizziness due to a deficiency of Heart-Blood.

Heart-8
Fire Point
On the palm of the hand, between the fourth and fifth metacarpal bones, on the distal transverse crease ('heart line').
- Clears Heart-Fire and Heart Phlegm-Fire; calms the Mind; useful for mental agitation, insomnia and nightmares due to Fire and Phlegm-Fire in the Heart.

Heart-9
Wood Point
About 0.1 cun from the base of the little fingernail at the radial side.
- Clears Excess Heat from the Heart; calms hysteria.
- Helps restore consciousness; may be used in cases of delirium and fainting.

Heart Protector Channel

Heart Protector-5
Metal Point
3 cun directly above the midpoint of the transverse crease of the wrist, between the two tendons.
- Clears Phlegm and Phlegm-Fire from the Heart when it 'mists the orifices' of the Mind, causing problems such as mental confusion, impulsive behaviour and manic depression.
- Smoothes the flow of Ki in the Heart.

Heart Protector-6
2 cun directly above the midpoint of the transverse crease of the wrist, between the two tendons.
- Moves Ki and Blood in the Heart; opens the chest; useful for feelings of constriction or pain in the chest.
- Calms the Mind, allays frustration and stops pain; may be used in cases of pre-menstrual tension and menstrual pain.
- Descends 'rebellious Ki' in the Stomach; especially in cases of nausea and vomiting.

Kidney Channel

Kidney-1
Wood Point
On the sole of the foot, one-third the distance from the base of the 2nd toe to the back of the heel.
- Tonifies the Yin and clears Heat due to Yin deficiency; calms the Mind; may be used in cases of extreme fear and anxiety.
- Descends Internal Wind and Heat causing problems such as dizziness, high blood pressure and headache on the vortex of the head.
- Clears the brain and restores consciousness.

Kidney-3
Earth Point
At the midpoint between the medial malleolus of the ankle and the Achilles tendon.
- Tonifies the Yin, Yang and Essence of the Kidneys; strengthens the Original Ki; often useful in cases of chronic debility and impotence.
- Benefits the Uterus; may be used in cases of infertility and amenorrhoea (lack of periods).
- Strengthens the waist, lower back and knees.

Kidney-6
1 cun directly below the medial malleolous of the ankle.
- Nourishes Kidney-Yin; useful for moistening the intestines, the eyes and the throat.
- Calms the Mind due to Yin-deficiency; may be used for insomnia with feelings of heat at night.
- Cools the Blood; may be used for skin conditions characterized by redness and dryness.
- Nourishes the Uterus; often useful in the case of infertility.

Kidney-7
Metal point
On the medial aspect of the lower leg, 2 cun above Kidney-3.
- Strengthens Kidney-Yang; clears Dampness from the Lower Heater and removes oedema from the legs.
- Adjusts sweating; tonified, it will stop excessive sweating; dispersed, it will promote sweating.

Large Intestine Channel

Large Intestine-4
With the thumb and index finger stretched apart, it is slightly to the index finger side of the area between the 1st and 2nd metacarpal bones.
- Expels External Wind and promotes the descending function of the Lungs; useful for blocked sinuses, sneezing, coughs and colds.
- Strengthens the Defensive-Ki.

- Stops pain, especially in the face; may be used for toothache, sinusitis and headache on the front of the head.

CONTRAINDICATED IN PREGNANCY

Large Intestine-10
2 cun distal to Large Intestine-11 on the forearm.
- Invigorates the flow of Ki along the Channels of the forearm and hand; eliminates painful obstructions; may be used to relieve muscular spasm, paralysis and rheumatic pain.
- Tonifies Ki and Blood.

Large Intestine-11
Earth Point
With the anterior surface of the forearm across the chest, the point lies between the lateral end of the elbow crease and the lateral epicondyle of the humerus.
- Disperses External Wind, especially Wind-Heat.
- Clears both Heat and Damp-Heat from the body; useful in cases of mucus colitis.
- Cools the Blood and benefits the skin; useful in cases of eczema and psoriasis.
- Benefits the sinews and joints; may be used for rheumatism and arthritis, especially when the arms and shoulders are affected.
- Helps to lower blood pressure.

Large Intestine-20
0.5 cun lateral to the nostril, in the nasolabial sulcus.
- Disperses External Wind from the face; benefits the nose; useful in cases of sneezing, nasal congestion and sinusitis.
- Local Tsubo for all nose problems; may be used to treat recurring nosebleeds.

Liver Channel

Liver-2
Fire Point
In the web between the first and second toes.
- Sedates Liver-Fire and Liver-Yang; often useful in cases of headache, red eyes, insomnia and excessive anger.
- Subdues Internal Wind; may be used in cases of dizziness and vertigo.
- Cools the Blood; often useful in cases of excessively heavy menstruation.

Liver-3
Earth Point
On the foot, 1.5–2 cun above the web between the first and second toes.
- Sedates rising Liver-Yang in a more gentle way than Liver-2; may be used in cases of migraine.

- Smoothes the flow of Liver-Ki, especially when stagnant Ki affects the epigastrium, abdomen and head.
- Calms the Mind; useful for treating irritability, frustration and tension.

Liver-4
Metal Point
At the anterior flexure of the ankle, between the tendons of the tibialis anterior and extensor hallucis longus.

- Smoothes the flow of Liver-Ki in the Lower Heater, especially in the genital and urinary area; may be used for swelling in the lower abdomen, painful urination and impotence.

Liver-8
Water Point
With the knee flexed, it is in the depression at the medial end of the transverse crease on the medial aspect of the knee, posterior to the medial condyle of the tibia.

- Eliminates Dampness from the Lower Heater, especially the Bladder; often useful in cases of urethritis, cystitis and leukorrhoea.
- Tonifies Liver-Blood.
- Relaxes the tendons.

Liver-13
Collecting (Bo) Point of the Spleen
At the anterior end of the eleventh rib.

- Smoothes the flow of Liver-Ki, especially when it 'invades' the Spleen and Stomach; often useful for abdominal swelling, flatulence and loose stools.
- Has a secondary effect of strengthening the Spleen.

Liver-14
Collecting (Bo) Point of the Liver
On the inferior edge of the thoracic cage, on the paramedian nipple line.

- Smoothes the flow of Liver-Ki, especially when it 'invades' the Stomach; often useful for epigastric swelling, belching and nausea.
- Smoothes the flow of Liver-Ki in the chest; indicated in cases of Ki stagnation in the chest causing a sense of constriction or fullness and difficult breathing.
- Moves and cools the Blood.

Lung Channel

Lung-1
Front Collecting (Bo) Point of the Lungs
Approximately 1 cun below the lateral end of the clavicle in the lateral part of the 1st intercostal space.

- Circulates and helps descend Lung-Ki; eliminates Heat and Phlegm from the chest; may be used for Full conditions of the Lungs involving cough, congestion and pain.
- Moves Blood in the chest.

Lung-5
Water point
On the transverse crease of the elbow, approximately 1 cun lateral to the tendon of the biceps muscle.
- Clears Heat from the Lungs; useful in cases of cough and bronchitis with yellow mucus and thirst.
- Dispels both Phlegm-Heat and Phlegm-Cold from the Lungs; may be used for congestion involving either yellow or white sputum.
- Alleviates pain in the elbow and forearm.

Lung-7
Proximal to the styloid process of the radius, 1.5 cun above the transverse crease of the wrist.
- Promotes the dispersing and descending of Lung-Ki; often useful in cases of coughing and asthma.
- Disperses External Wind, especially Wind-Cold; promotes sweating; an important Tsubo for colds and flu.
- Clears the nose; useful for blocked sinuses, sneezing and loss of sense of smell.
- Stimulates the free passage of fluids and benefits the Bladder; often useful in cases of oedema and urinary retention.

Lung-9
Earth Point
On the transverse crease of the wrist, between the radius and scaphoid bones.
- Tonifies Lung-Ki; may be used when there is lethargy, pallor, shallow breathing and a weak voice.
- Strengthens Gathering-Ki (see p.129); helps the Heart to circulate the Blood.
- Tonifies Lung-Yin; often useful for a dry cough, thirst, feelings of Heat and blood in the sputum.
- Clears Phlegm from the Lungs.

Lung-10
Fire Point
At the midpoint on the thenar surface of the 1st metacarpus.
- Disperses Heat from the Lungs; cools the throat; useful for a sore, inflamed throat.

Lung-11
Wood Point
Approximately 0.1 cun from the base of the cuticle on the inside of the thumb.
- Disperses External Wind-Heat; useful in cases of very high fever.

- Cools the throat; may be used for a sore throat due to an invasion of Wind-Heat.
- Expels Internal Wind and restores consciousness.

Spleen Channel

Spleen-3
Earth Point
On the posterior, inferior aspect at the head of the 1st metatarsal bone.
- Tonifies the Spleen; transforms Dampness; may be used for abdominal bloating, loose stools, diarrhoea, and both physical and mental sluggishness.

Spleen-6
Meeting Point of the Spleen, Liver and Kidney Channels
At the posterior margin of the tibia, 3 cun directly above the medial malleolus of the ankle.
- Tonifies the Spleen; useful for deficiency of Ki and Blood due to Spleen weakness.
- Clears Dampness due to impairment of the Spleen's function of transformation and transportation, especially in the Lower Heater; useful in cases of cystitis and leukorrhoea.
- Helps smooth the flow of Liver-Ki; stops pain; may be used for pre-menstrual tension and painful periods.
- Calms the mind when there is stagnant Ki; good for relieving frustration and tension.
- Moves the Blood; especially when stagnant Blood causes gynaecological problems such as dysmenorrhoea (painful periods) with the presence of clots in the menstrual blood.
- Benefits the Uterus; regulates menstruation.
- Nourishes Kidney-Yin; useful in cases of a dry mouth at night, thirst and hot flushes.

CONTRAINDICATED IN PREGNANCY

Spleen-9
Water Point
On the posterior edge of the tibia, at the inferior margin of the medial condyle of the tibia, 13 cun proximal to the prominence of the medial malleolus.
- Clears Dampness from the Lower Heater and Bladder in particular; useful in cases of cystitis, cloudy urine, mucus in the stools and leukorrhoea.

Spleen-10
2 cun above the superior medial border of the kneecap, on the medial margin of the vastus medialis muscle of the thigh.
- Cools the Blood; may be used to clear Heat from the Blood causing skin diseases such as psoriasis, and excessive menstrual bleeding.

- Moves the Blood and regulates menstruation; useful in cases of dysmenorrhoea due to stagnation of Blood.

Stomach Channel

Stomach-21
4 cun above the navel and 2 cun lateral to the median line.
- Descends 'Rebellious Ki' in the Stomach causing hiccups, belching, acid reflux (heartburn) and nausea; especially good for acute conditions.
- Clears Heat from the Stomach.

Stomach-25
Front Collecting (Bo) Point of the Large Intestines
2 cun directly lateral to the navel.
- Moves Ki in the Intestines and Stomach; useful in cases of abdominal swelling and constipation, especially when there is retention of food.
- Clears Heat from the Intestines and Stomach; helps resolve Stomach Phlegm-Fire; may be used for foul-smelling diarrhoea, burning pain and manic behaviour involving Phlegm-Fire.

Stomach-36
Earth Point
13 cun proximal to the prominence of the lateral malleolus, 3 cun below the lateral 'eye' of the knee, lateral to the edge of the tibia.
- Tonifies the Ki and Blood of the entire body; strengthens the Stomach and Spleen; may be used for chronic debility, weak Defensive Ki, abdominal distension, poor digestion and anaemia.
- Warms the Yang (especially with moxibustion) and disperses Cold, Wind and Damp; may be used to promote sweating and expel External Wind-Cold and Wind-Damp from the muscles and joints. (N.B. the Tsubo should first be dispersed to eliminate the External factor; then treated with moxibustion in order to warm.)
- Adjusts the function of the Intestines; may be used for diarrhoea or constipation due to deficiency.

Stomach-40
On the lower leg, 8 cun above the lateral malleolus of the ankle and 1 cun lateral to the edge of the tibia.
- The main Tsubo to eliminate Phlegm and Dampness from the body; may be used for excessive catarrh production, a 'wheezing' chest and asthma; for cloudy urine and mucus in the stools; for lumps and cysts; and for Phlegm 'misting the orifices' of the Mind, creating mental confusion and obsessiveness.
- Clears Heat from the Stomach and pacifies the Stomach; often useful in the case of nervous indigestion.
- Calms the Mind; eases anxiety and worry.

Stomach-44
Water point
At the proximal end of the web between the second and third toes.
- Moves Stomach-Ki and eliminates 'Retention of Food', clears Stomach-Heat; may be used for feelings of fullness, pain or burning in the epigastrium, as well as for flatulence and acid reflux (heartburn).
- Eliminates Heat, obstruction and Wind from the face, especially along the Stomach Channel; often useful in cases of nosebleed, bleeding gums, toothache and facial neuralgia.
- Moves Ki and relieves fullness and pain in the Intestines.

Triple Heater

Triple Heater-5
2 cun above the transverse crease on the posterior surface of the forearm, between the ulna and radius.
- Disperses External Wind-Heat; useful in cases of feverishness, headache and sore throat due to an invasion of Wind-Heat.
- Benefits the ears; may be used in cases of earache due to External Wind-Heat or hearing problems caused by rising Liver-Yang and Liver-Fire.
- Relieves pain along the Triple Heater Channel; may be used for painful obstructions of the neck, shoulders and arms; eases headaches on the sides of the head.

Triple Heater-6
Fire Point
3 cun above the transverse crease on the posterior surface of the forearm, 1 cun above Triple Heater-5.
- Moves Ki in all three Heaters, but mainly in the Intestines and flanks; smoothes the flow of Liver-Ki; may be used in cases of constipation or flank pain involving stagnant Liver-Ki.
- Clears Heat from all three Heaters; clears Wind-Heat from the Blood causing sudden rashes.

Triple Heater-23
In the depression at the lateral end of the eyebrow.
- Benefits the eyes; may be used as a local Tsubo for any problem affecting the eyes, especially when the Liver is involved.
- Eases pain in the sides of the face by eliminating obstruction and Wind along the Channel; useful in cases of headache on the temples, facial paralysis and dizziness.

Index